About this Booklet

Dental implant therapy has dramatically helped many people who are missing some or all of their teeth. Read this booklet for answers to the following questions and many more:

What are dental implants?
Are they for you?
How are they placed in your mouth?
What is the best way for you to take care of them?

Remember—the information given is *general*. You are a unique individual! Only your dentist can adapt this information to fit your situation.

WHAT IS AN IMPLANT?

An implant is an artificial object that replaces a missing body part. An implant is placed *inside* the body and acts almost like the missing body part. For instance, two common examples of implants are a hip joint replacement and a shoulder joint replacement. A mechanical ball and socket can replace a worn-out hip joint so that the leg can move back and forth. In the same way, a mechanical ball and socket can replace a worn-out shoulder joint.

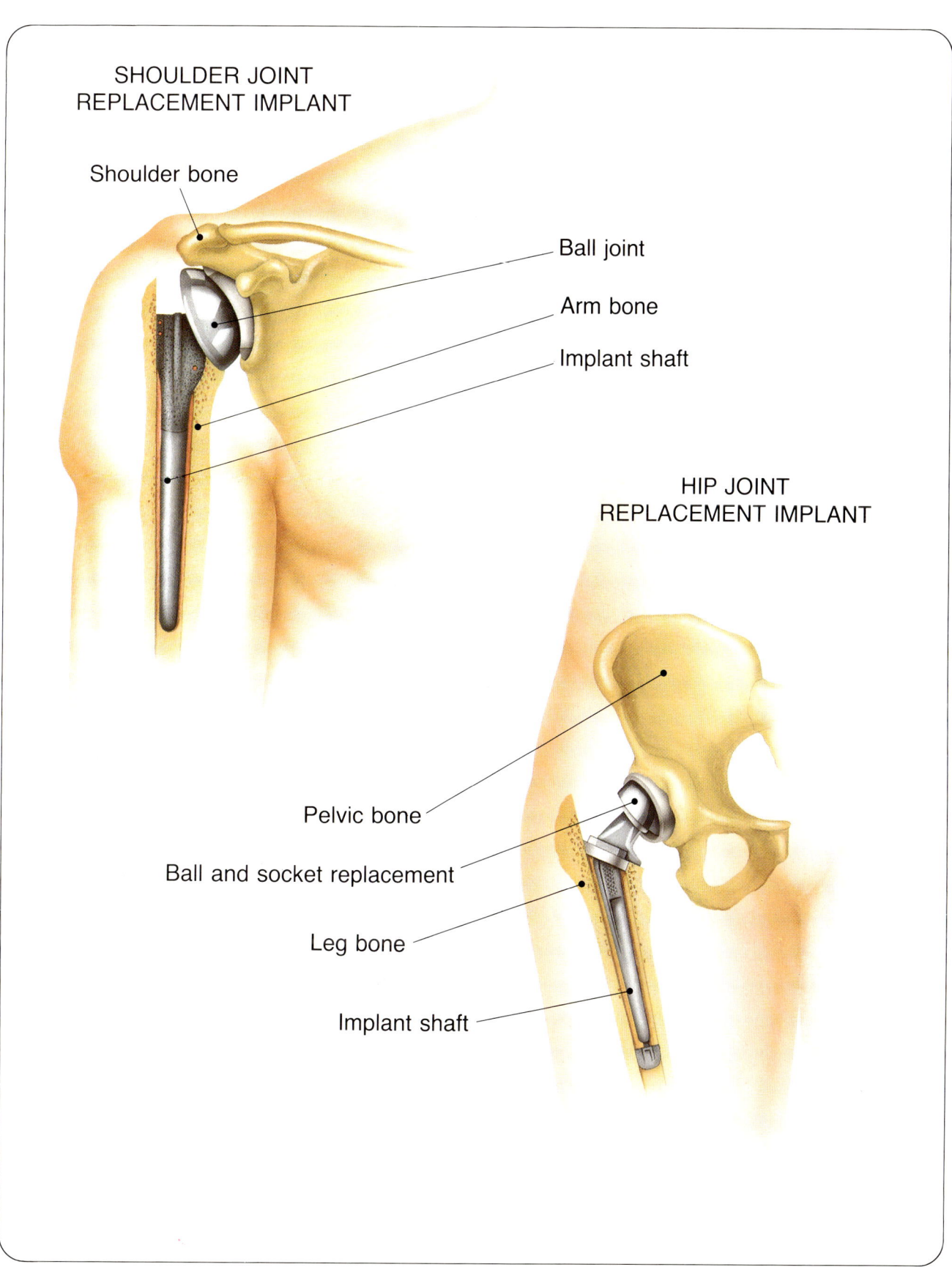

WHAT IS A DENTAL IMPLANT?

Another type of implant is a **dental implant.** In this case, when natural teeth are missing from the mouth, devices to replace the **root portion** of teeth are put into the bone and gums of the mouth. Artificial teeth are then fixed onto these devices. Dental implants allow people who are missing teeth to be able to chew well and comfortably.

This booklet will help you understand the benefits and risks involved with dental implants. Your dentist can give you complete information on your specific situation and help you decide if dental implants are for you.

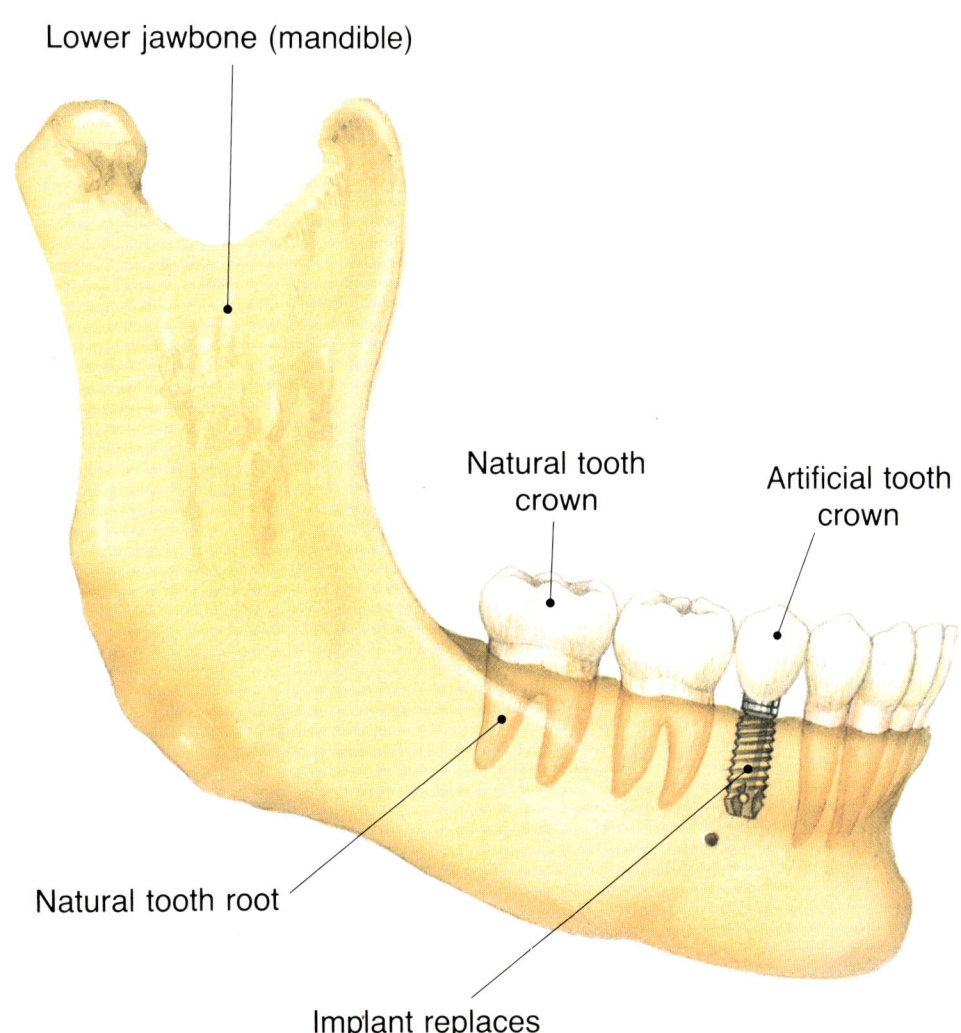

WHAT MOUTH CONDITIONS MIGHT REQUIRE A DENTAL IMPLANT?

If you are missing a tooth or teeth, or even parts of your jaw, these could be replaced with dental implants. First, there are a few very important factors that must be considered.

Experiments and practical experience have shown that implants work best when there is enough dense, healthy jawbone in a mouth that will support an implant.

Healthy, disease-free gum tissues are also necessary. The long-term success of a dental implant depends upon keeping the gums and bone around the implant healthy. People who have implants must keep them clean and should return regularly to their dentist for checkups, because any problems that might threaten the health of the implant must be corrected.

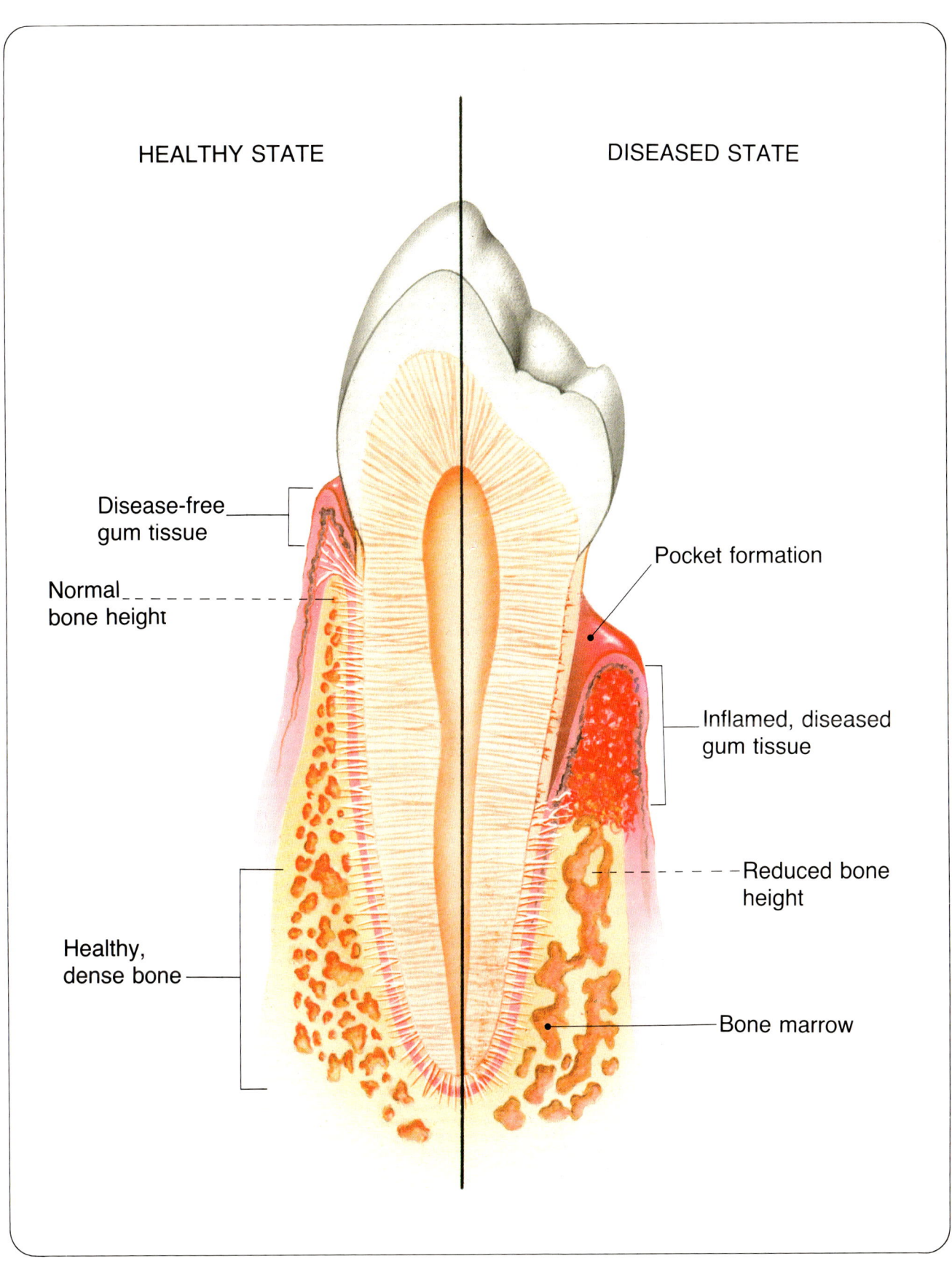

WHO SHOULD *NOT* HAVE DENTAL IMPLANTS?

If you have any of the following conditions, dental implant therapy may not be for you.

Crippling or uncontrolled disease

Conditions that affect the body's ability to heal and repair itself may have a negative effect on the placement and health of an implant. Persons with diseases (such as diabetes) that are not under control are not good candidates for dental implants because the uncontrolled disease keeps the body from healing itself normally. However, a diabetic person under proper control by a doctor could be treated successfully with implants.

Other diseases such as leukemia or hyperparathyroidism (abnormal activity of the parathyroid glands) also may affect the outcome of implant treatment. Persons who are having chemotherapy or radiation therapy for cancer should not have treatment procedures that are advantageous but not urgent (such as dental implants) until cancer treatment is completed and the doctor says it is safe to proceed. If you have any questions about how your general health might affect dental implants in your mouth, you and your dentist should discuss this with your doctor.

Pregnancy

Women who are pregnant should not undergo any treatment such as dental implants until after the first three months of their pregnancy. It is best to wait until after delivery to start dental implant treatment.

Psychiatric or emotional treatment

People with psychiatric disorders such as chronic depression or personality changes requiring treatment, or people undergoing severe emotional stress should avoid situations that may complicate or disturb their lives. Dental implant therapy may place additional stress on persons who are unable to tolerate it. As with other diseases, open discussion of the problem should involve the patient, dentist, and doctor before implant treatment is considered.

Poor motivation to accept and follow needed treatment

For dental implants to be successful, you must be committed to following all the necessary steps before, during, and long after treatment. People who are not able or not willing to undergo the necessary treatment, or to take care of their new teeth on a regular basis, should not consider implant therapy.

Lack of muscular coordination to manage oral hygiene procedures

To keep the bone and gums around dental implants healthy, you must carefully clean the implants. This means that you must be able to handle a toothbrush, dental floss, or other cleaning tools to remove food and plaque. Persons with severe arthritis or other handicaps that affect the hands and arms may not be good candidates for implant treatment.

ARE DENTAL IMPLANTS FOR ME?

- Are you missing all natural teeth in one or both jaws?

- Are you missing one or more teeth in a jaw?

- Are you having difficulty wearing a regular removable denture because you gag, find the denture is too bulky, feel pain, or generally dislike something movable in the mouth?

- Do you have an oral defect or missing mouth part because of an injury, surgery to treat disease, or birth defect?

If you answered yes to any of the above conditions or preferences, you may be a candidate for dental implants.

Your age generally will not prevent the placement or use of dental implants. However, pre-adolescent or very elderly persons may not be good candidates for treatment.

Missing some teeth
(partially edentulous)

Missing all natural teeth
(completely edentulous)

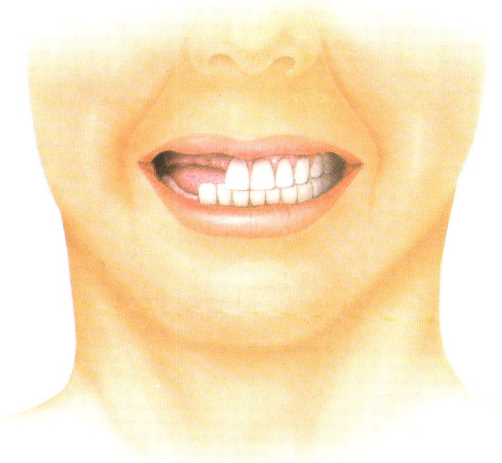
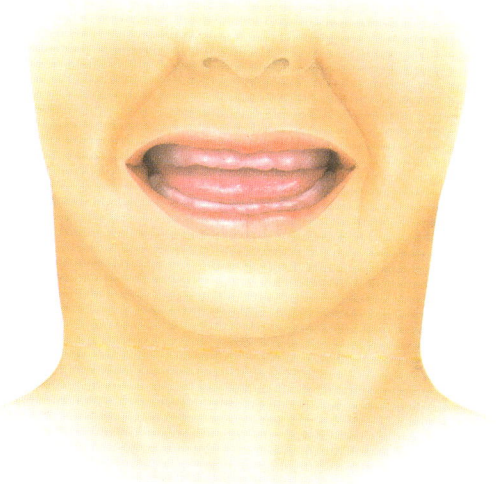

Oral defect
(cleft palate)

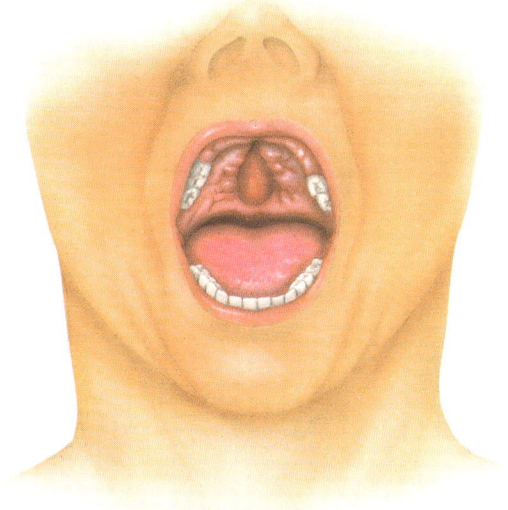

ARE THERE ANY RISKS TO MY HEALTH WITH IMPLANT TREATMENT?

Some health factors are important when considering dental implants:

Surgery or anesthetic

Usual precautions associated with a local or general anesthetic must be taken. Sometimes an opening into the sinus cavity above the upper teeth or a nerve injury can occur. These incidents seldom result in permanent damage.

Psychological

People who experience abnormal psychologic stresses or do not motivate well may have problems with surgery and may not be able or willing to follow oral hygiene instructions. However, persons who avoid contact with other people because they are concerned about their missing or unattractive teeth may be helped.

Medical

There are some temporary conditions that can result from implant placement: pain and swelling of gums, lip, or tongue, speech problems, and inflammation (heat, redness, swelling, and pain) of the gums. Possible long-term difficulties may include nerve injury, bone loss if the implants fail, overgrowth of gums, and mouth or general bacterial infection. For those people who have other body part replacements or heart valve problems, endocarditis (inflammation of the inside lining of the heart) or infection may be a risk.

WHO SHOULD PLACE IMPLANTS?

Implant treatment is a highly technical, complex form of dentistry. It is not a type of treatment that all dentists can or want to provide. Ask your dentist about his or her training and experience with dental implants. If you are considering this type of treatment and your dentist does not work with implants, he or she may be able to refer you to someone with the necessary training and experience.

Implant treatment may be provided in several ways.

1. Implants can be placed in your jaw by a team of dental specialists. This might include an oral surgeon or a periodontist who performs the surgical procedures, and a prosthodontist or a restorative dentist who designs and makes the teeth.
2. A dentist who has had extensive implant and dental training and limits his or her practice to implants may both perform the surgery and make the teeth.
3. A general dentist with particular knowledge, skills, and training may include implant procedures in his or her practice and perform all the procedures.

A team approach (several doctors) to treatment is generally preferred, because all members of the team see the patient for consultation, examination, and planning before any treatment is started.

WHAT ARE THE TYPES OF IMPLANTS?
WHICH IMPLANT IS BEST FOR ME?

There are three types of implants, and they can be described according to their shape and how they are attached to the jaws.

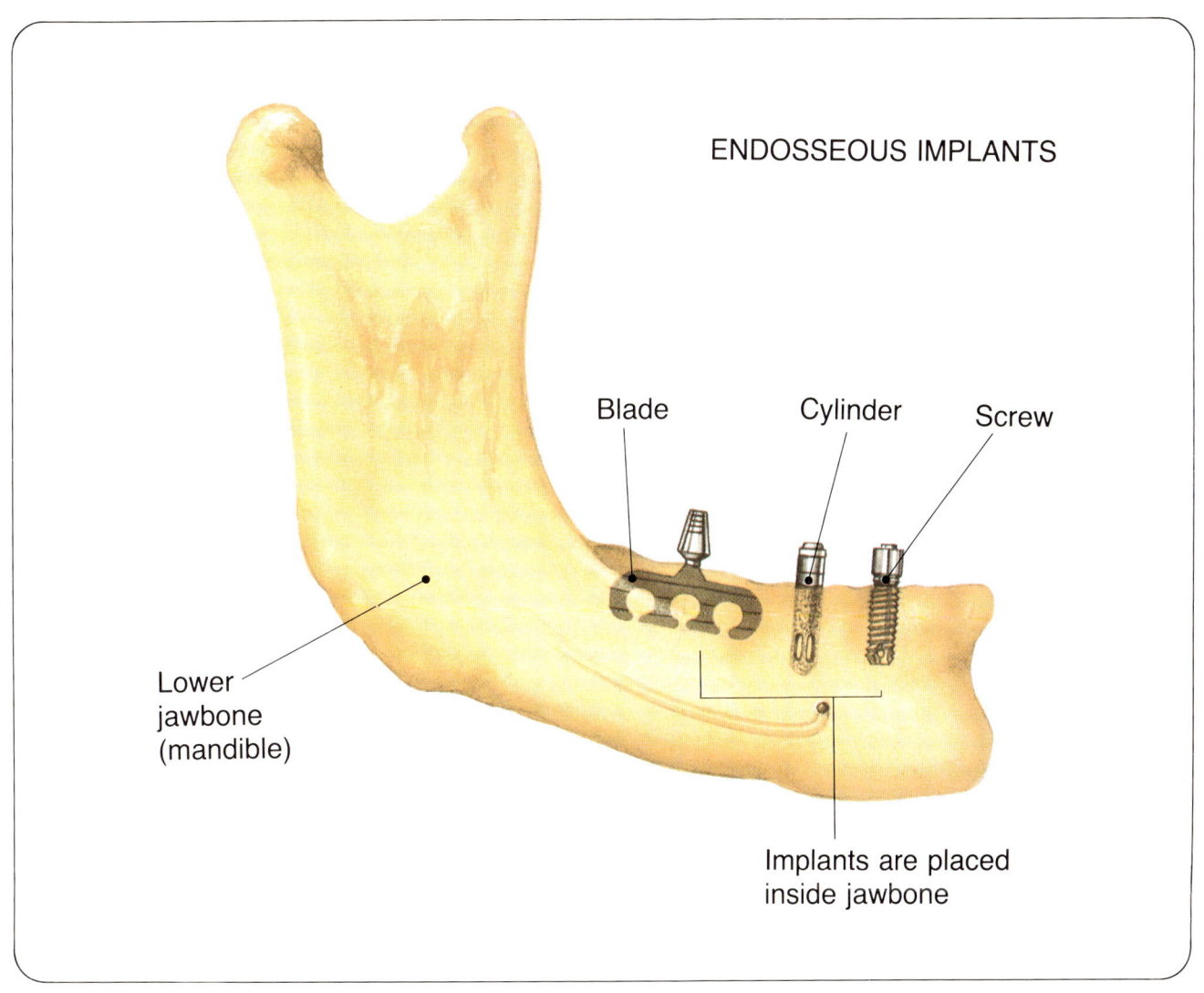

ENDOSSEOUS (en-dosś-ee-us)—"*within* the bone"

These implants are usually shaped like a screw or cylinder and are made either of metal, metal covered with ceramic, or ceramic material. They are placed *within* the jawbone. There are also blade-shaped endosseous implants.

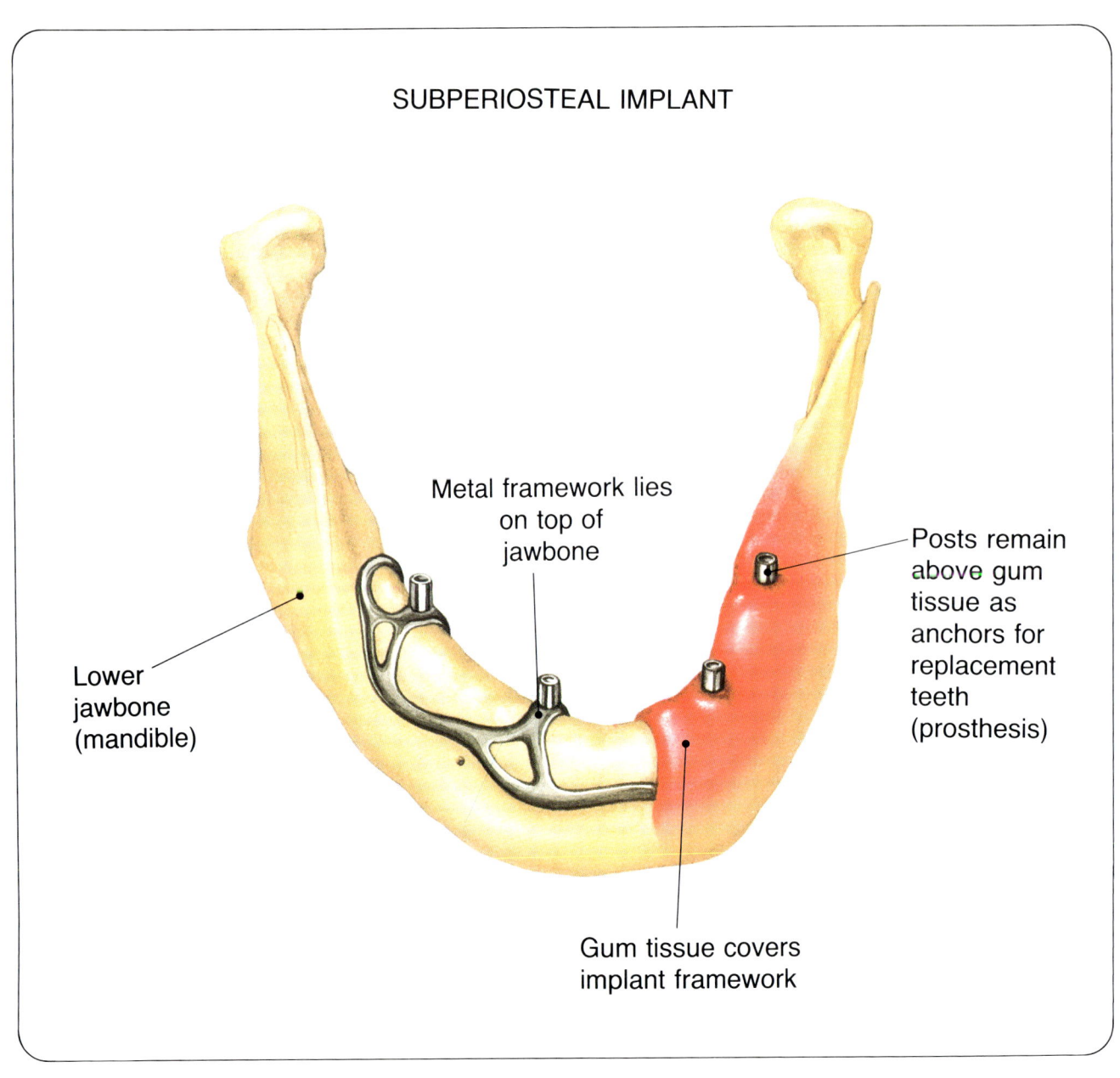

SUBPERIOSTEAL (sub-pear-ee-osś-tee-al)— "*on top* of the bone"

These implants consist of a metal framework that attaches *on top* of the jawbone but underneath the gum tissue.

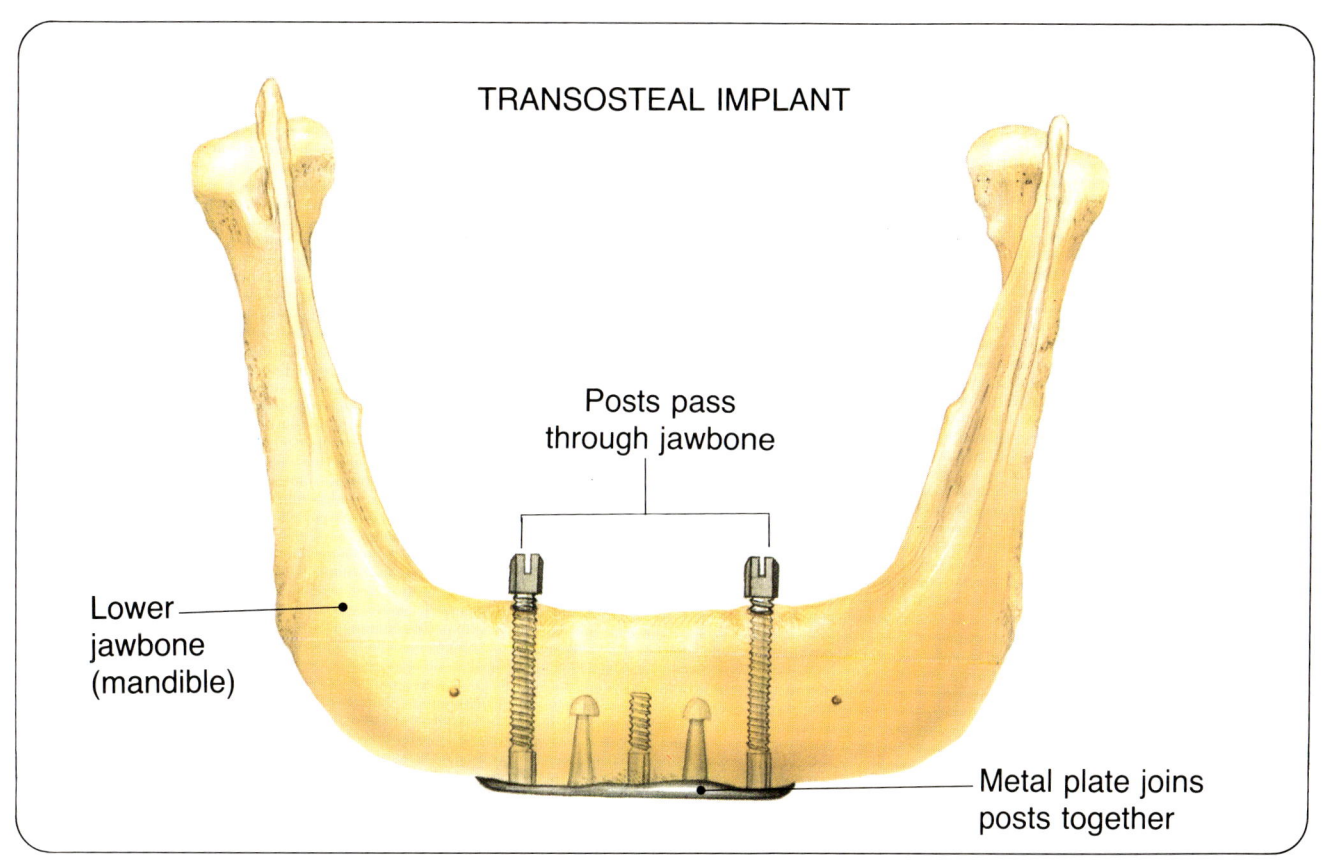

TRANSOSTEAL (trans-osś-tee-al)—*"through the bone"*

These implants are either a metal pin or a U-shaped frame that passes *through* the jawbone and the gum tissue, into the mouth.

The dental specialist or general dentist chooses the type, size, and design of dental implant. This choice is made according to where the implant will be placed, what kind of bone and how much bone is available, and the design of the tooth or teeth that will be placed on the implant(s). Your dentist will determine which type is best suited to your needs.

WHAT IS OSSEOINTEGRATION?

When dental implants that have been placed in your jawbone are successful, **osseointegration** occurs. This term means **bone connection.** The metal or ceramic part of the implant is placed into your jawbone, then the bone actually attaches itself directly to the implant, growing all around it and supporting it firmly.

Some implant systems encourage a soft tissue scar layer between the implant and bone; it is suggested that this scar tissue serves like a ligament in connecting a natural tooth root to its bony socket. However, this theory has not been scientifically proven. In addition, a scar layer contributes to implant movement, permitting undesirable communication between bone and the mouth, and does not react well to biting forces.

Scientific data do tell us that implant systems based on osseointegration are predictable and highly successful. Your dentist can discuss this with you.

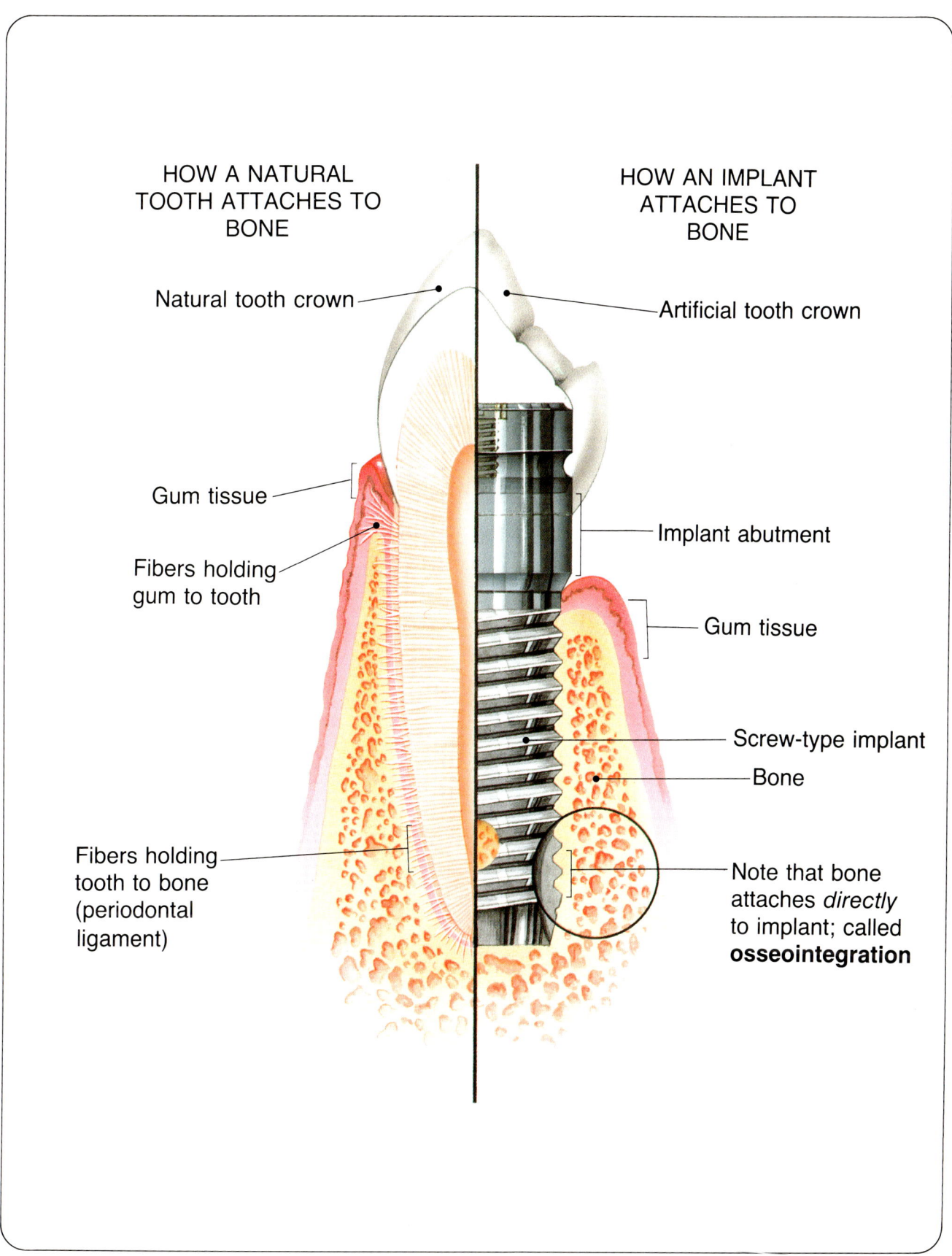

HOW LONG WILL DENTAL IMPLANTS LAST?

With advances in the science of implant dentistry, you can now expect that most implants will function indefinitely. However, like any dental restoration, the teeth may wear or break and need to be repaired or replaced.

COST

After you have been examined by your dentist and before you make any decision on implant treatment, you must consider cost. Just like any complicated and time-consuming medical or dental procedure, implant treatment is moderately expensive. You should be aware of *all* the costs involved. If you will be treated by a team of dentists, make sure that you receive cost estimates from each one involved. For example, if an oral surgeon is placing the implants into your jaw and a prosthodontist or your personal dentist is going to make the restoration (prosthesis) to replace the teeth, you should get cost estimates from both.

If you have dental insurance, you or your dentist should contact the insurance company *before* you start treatment to find out whether or how much of the treatment might be covered. Insurance policies vary in their coverage of elective procedures such as implants. It is important that, before you agree to proceed, you fully understand how much your insurance company will pay and how much you yourself will have to pay.

WHAT IS A TYPICAL COURSE OF IMPLANT TREATMENT?

On the following pages, a description will be given of how implants are placed in the mouth. The type of implant shown will be the *endosseous* implant, because it is the most common and probably the most successful type of implant used today. Treatment for your individual situation may vary, and your dentist will discuss this with you.

TIMETABLE OF A TYPICAL COURSE OF IMPLANT TREATMENT
(for a fixed prosthesis)

Examination and Diagnosis

Within 6 months before surgery	X-rays Other tests Impressions

Stage 1 Surgery

Date of surgery	Implants placed in jaw
4–5 days after surgery	Swelling disappears
7 days after surgery	Old denture is lined with soft material for continued wearing
10–14 days after surgery	Sutures dissolve or are removed
4–6 weeks after surgery	You must eat a soft diet during this time period
3–6 months after surgery	Healing is completed

Stage 2 Surgery

Day of surgery	Implants uncovered Osseointegration checked Abutments placed Healing caps or revised denture placed X-rays to check implant-abutment connection
4–5 days after surgery	Impressions of mouth made
10–14 days after surgery	Sutures dissolve or are removed

Restorative Treatment

1 month after Stage 2 Surgery	New prosthesis is completed Temporary seating of new teeth on implant abutments Final attachment of prosthesis

Follow-up Care

1 month, 3 months, and 6 months after Restorative Treatment (and yearly thereafter)	Follow-up examinations

Examination and diagnosis

When you first see your dentist to talk about the possibility of implant therapy, your mouth will be thoroughly examined. X-rays will be taken of your head, jaw, and teeth so your dentist can determine the type, amount, and location of bone that is available. You may have to undergo other tests to check blood characteristics, heart function, lung condition, and general health status.

X-ray unit
Jaw positioner

R
L

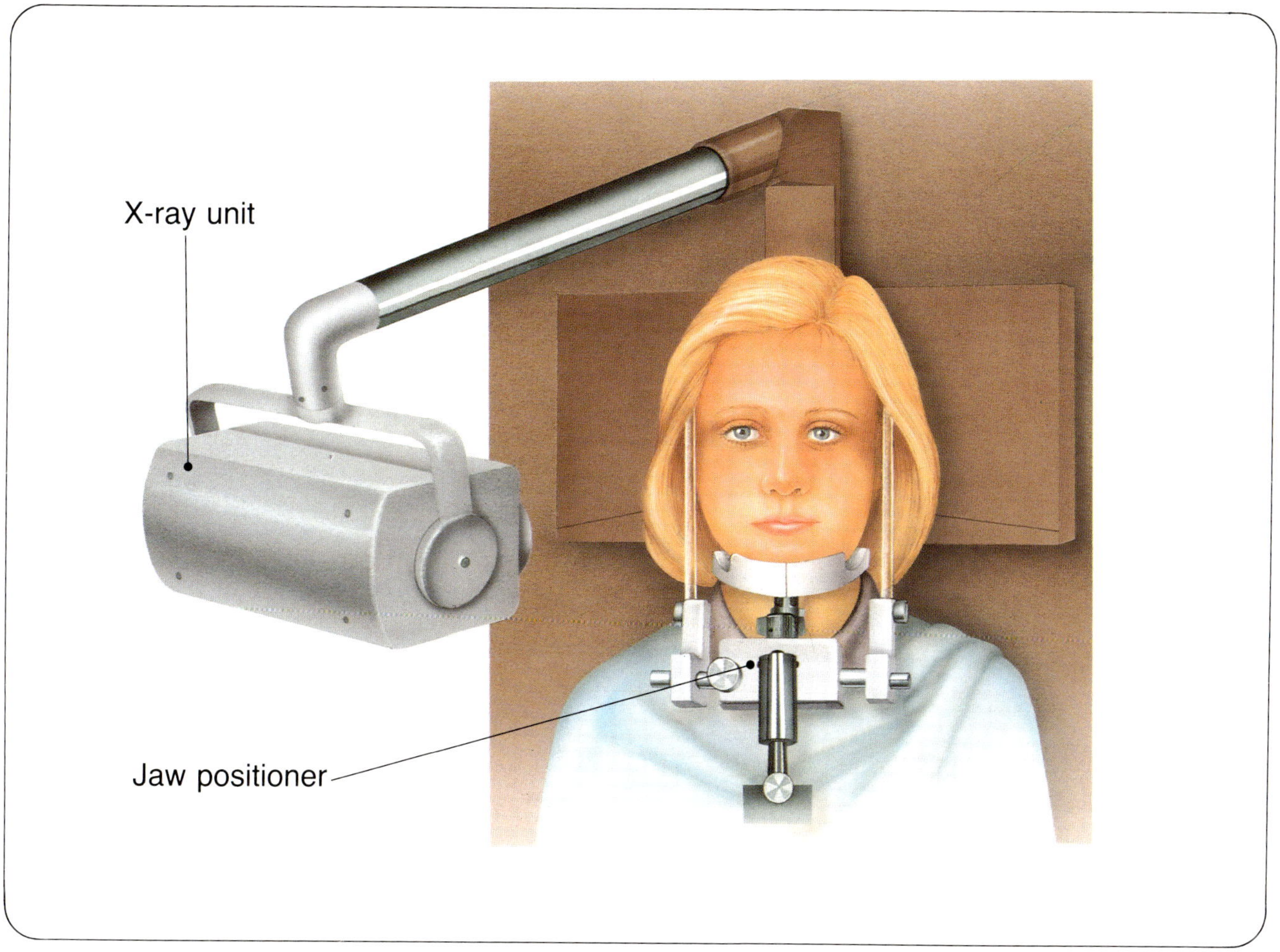

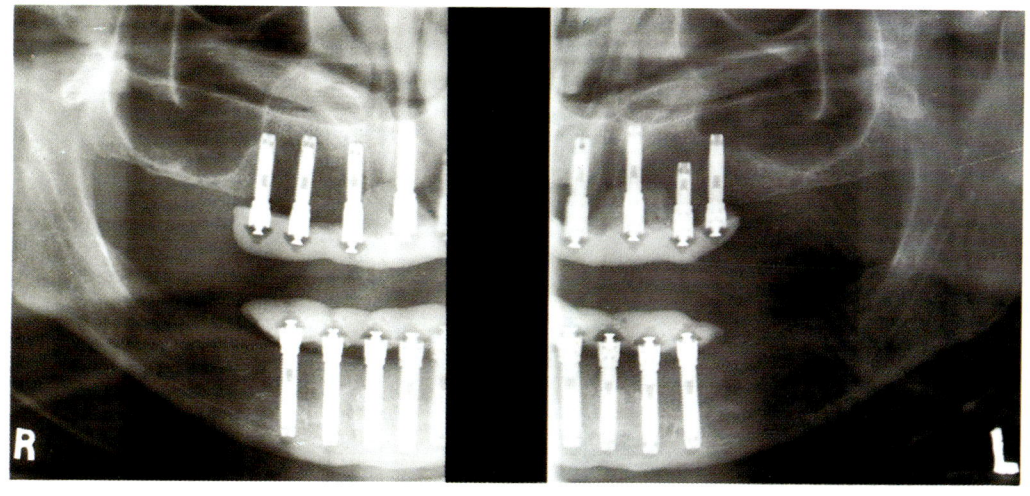

Impressions (molds) of the teeth and jaws are also necessary. Using these impressions, the dentist will then make plaster-like models so he or she can plan the treatment and make surgical guides. Such surgical guides help the surgeon to properly place the implants.

In addition, a psychological test may be given, which provides the dentist with insight into particular personality problems a person may have that could cause the treatment to be less successful than expected.

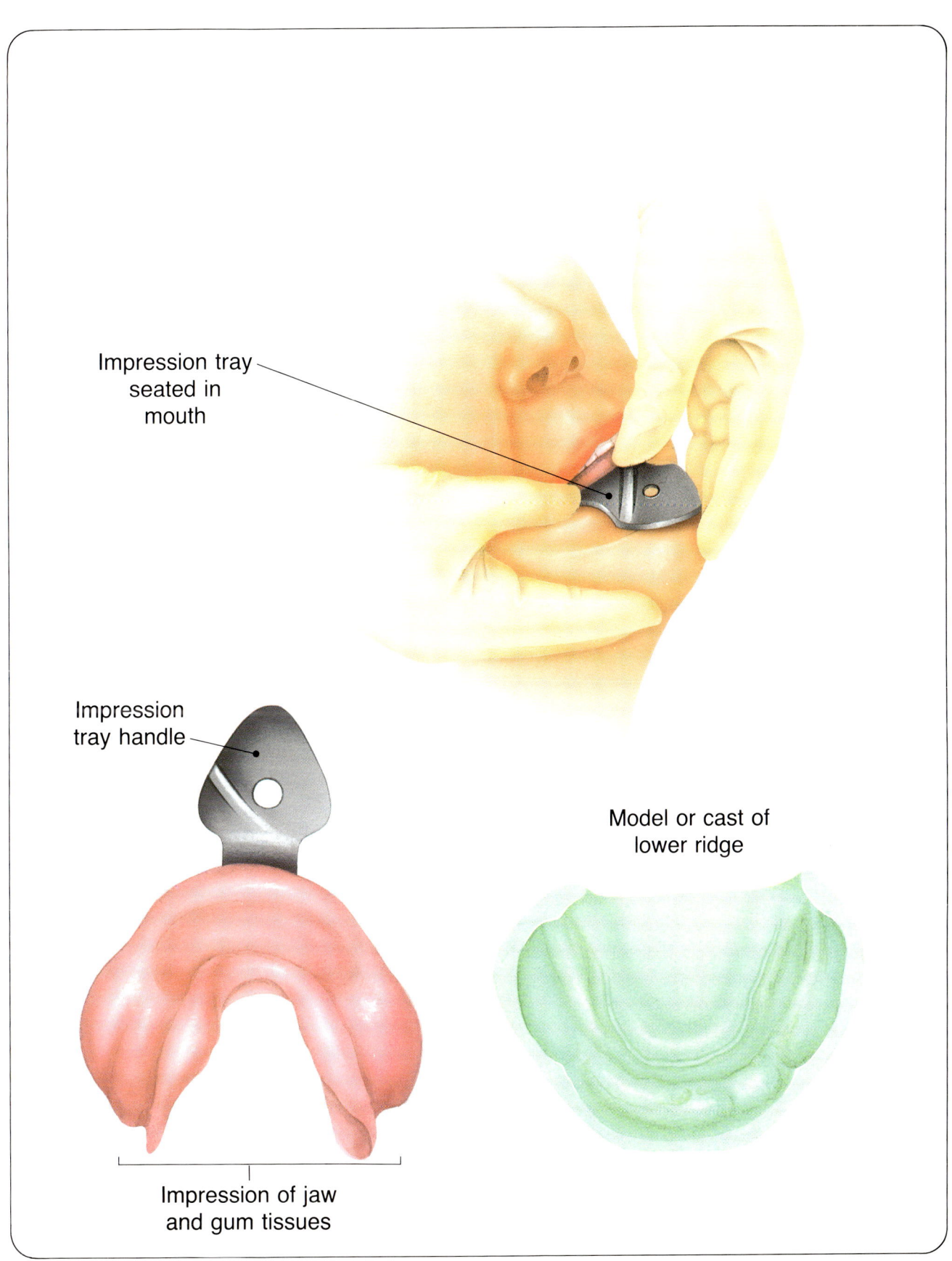

Surgery

Once you and your dentist have decided that implant therapy is right for you, the examination has been done, and your dentist has chosen the appropriate implant system, surgery will be scheduled. The surgical treatment is usually performed in two stages.

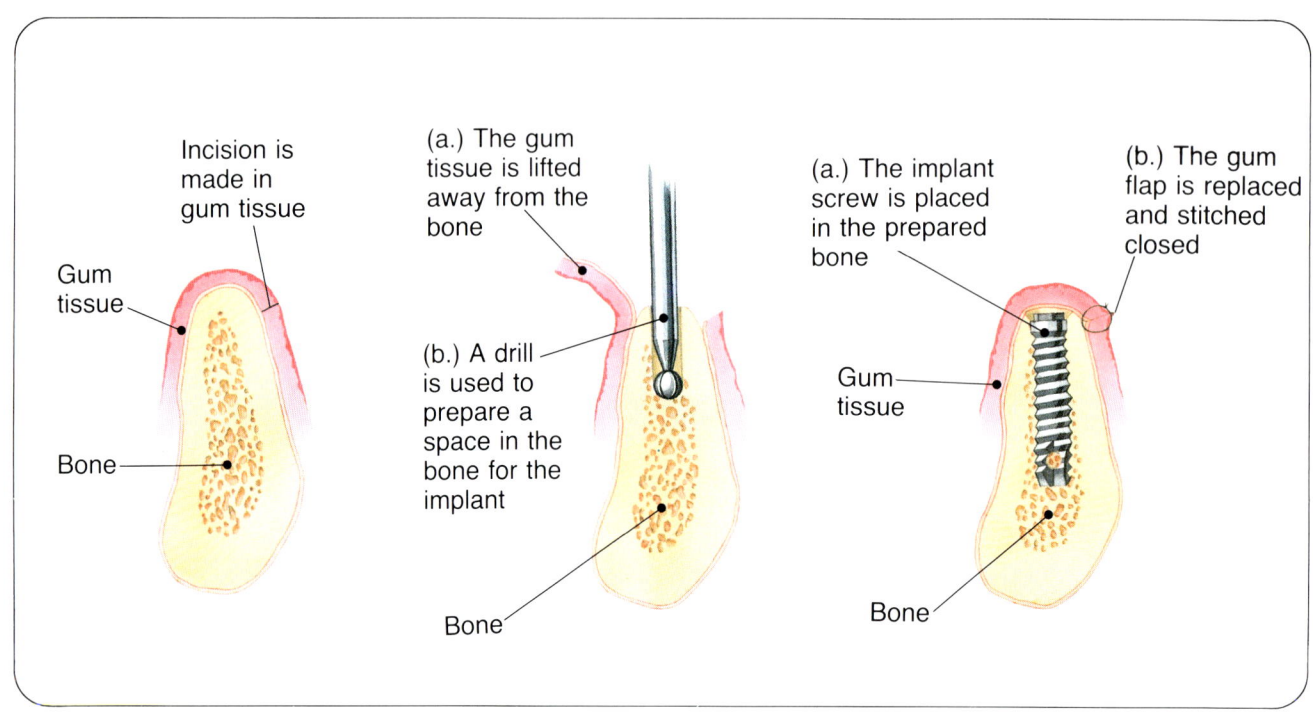

Stage 1 surgery

During the first operation, implants will be placed into the jawbone, underneath the gum tissues. They will stay "buried" under the gums for a healing time—from 3 to 6 months. (In the upper jaw and back part of the lower jaw, complete healing usually takes longer.) The surgery may be performed in an office setting with local anesthesia and perhaps mild sedation. Or, it can be performed in a hospital setting with general anesthesia. A sterile environment and gentle and cautious surgical procedure are essential to success. If the surgery is performed in a hospital, a one-night stay in the hospital after the procedures may be required.

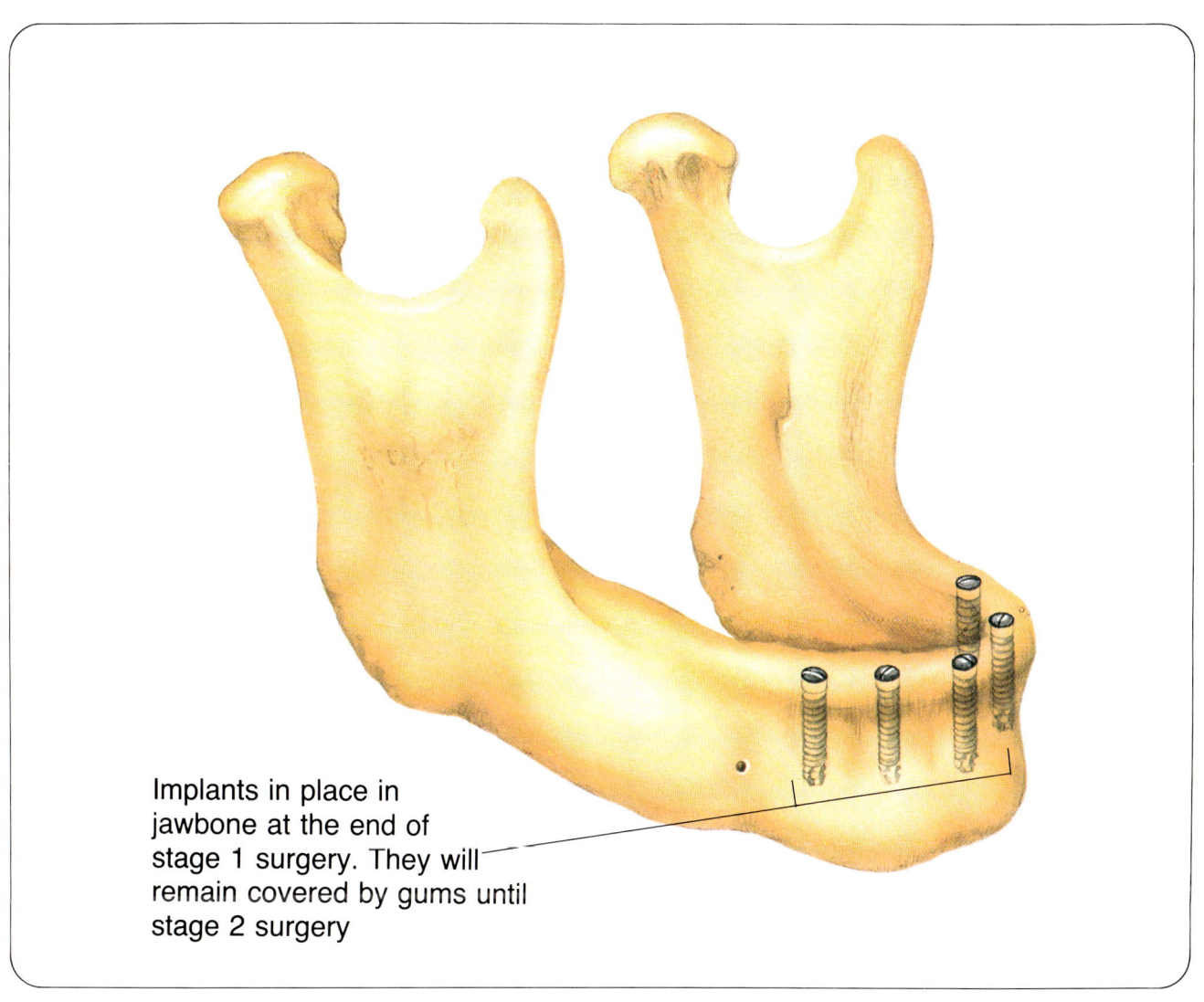

Implants in place in jawbone at the end of stage 1 surgery. They will remain covered by gums until stage 2 surgery

The day after surgery, you can expect some swelling of the gums in the area of implant placement. You may also be able to feel the sutures (stitches) that were used to close the incision. The gums may be discolored as they start to heal. When you had teeth removed before, you probably remember the pain experienced; the immediate discomfort at this time will likely be similar. Medication can be used to lessen the pain.

Within 4 to 5 days, the initial swelling will be gone and the surgical area will be less painful. The denture that you may have been wearing can be lined with a soft material and placed back in your mouth to improve your speech and appearance. You should be able to return to work or resume normal daily activities comfortably by this time.

If the stitches closing the wound have not come out on their own by this time, your dentist or surgeon may remove them after 10 to 14 days.

You must not use your denture to chew solid foods until your dentist says you can do so. The ability of your mouth to successfully accept implants depends on it not being disturbed during the first 4 to 6 weeks after surgery. A soft diet must be continued during this period.

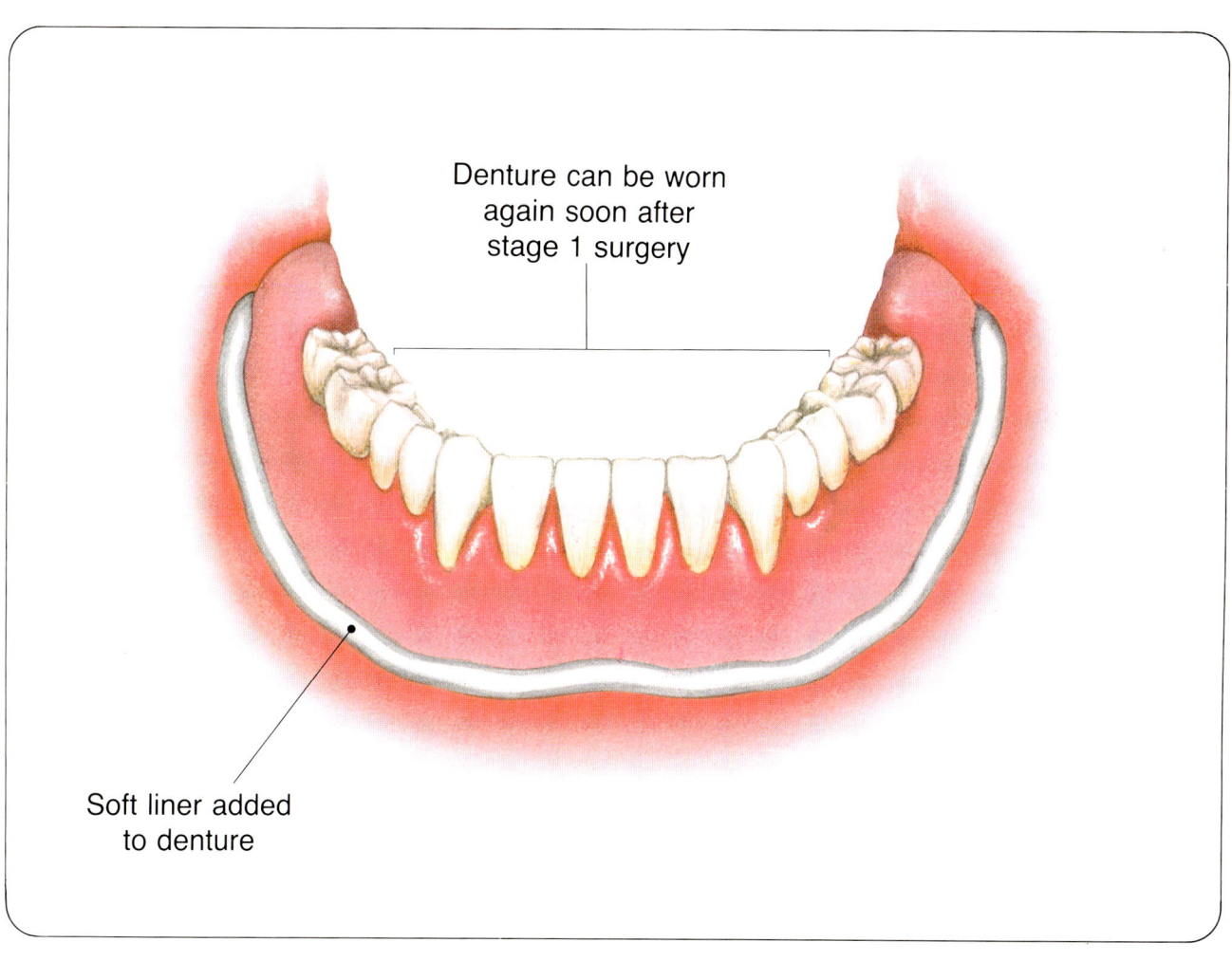

Stage 2 surgery

The second stage of surgical treatment can usually be done on an outpatient basis in an office setting 3 to 6 months after the implants have been placed. The surgeon will numb the area of previous surgery with a local anesthetic to make you more comfortable. The gum tissue is then opened in the area of the implants, to expose the implants. Extension posts, called **abutments,** are attached to the implants. (Eventually your new teeth will be attached to these abutments.) At this time, the implants are examined to be certain of their firmness and integration with the bone. The gums are then put back in place around the abutments and sutured (stitched) closed. Healing caps and a surgical packing or your old denture with a soft lining is then placed over the abutments to help the gum tissues heal and to lessen discomfort.

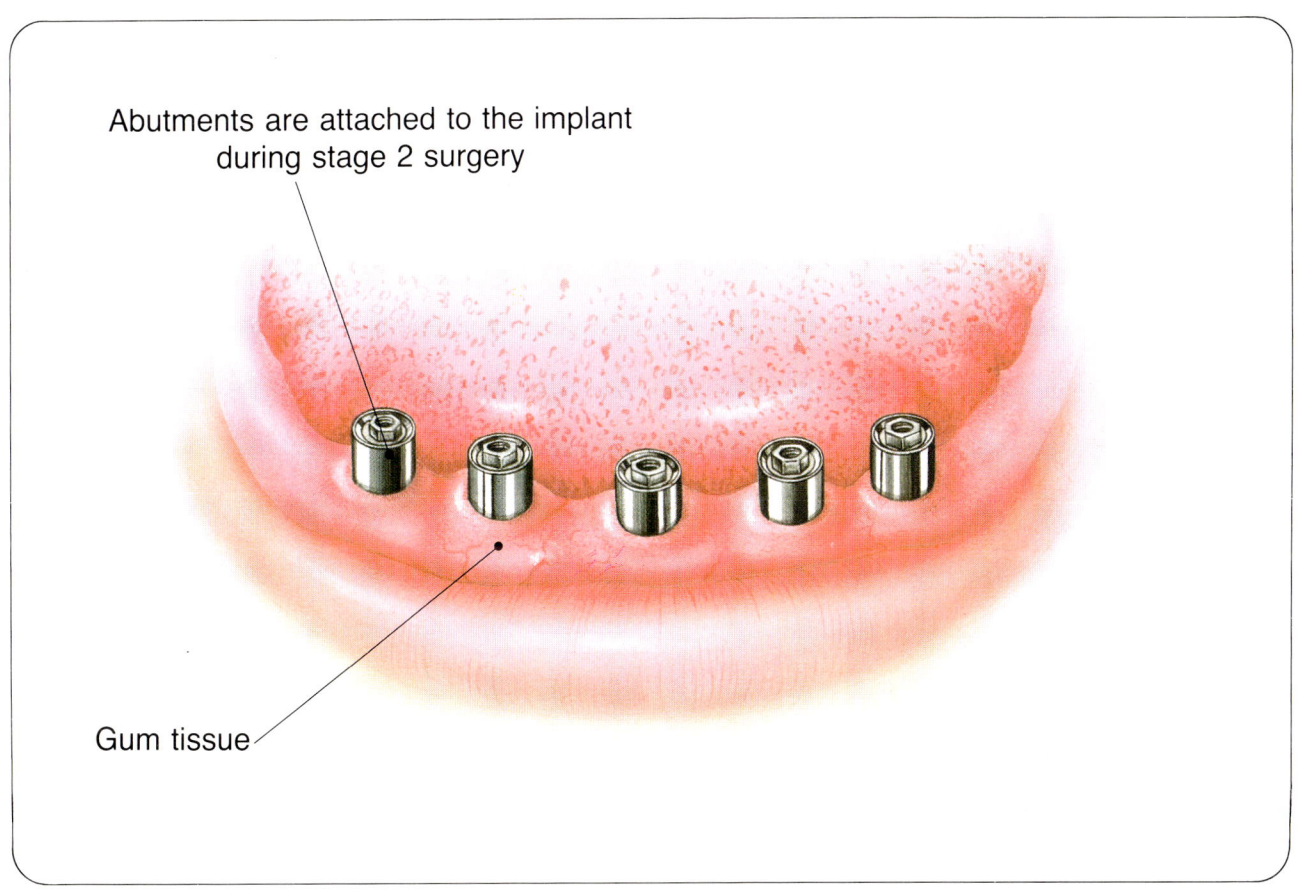

At this phase of treatment, the dentist will want to determine that **osseointegration** (see page 24) has been achieved and that the abutments are firmly and accurately attached to the implants. This requires an x-ray.

Several days after the abutments are attached, the surgical pack can be removed. If you are wearing a denture with a temporary lining, your dentist will continue to refit the lining to keep your mouth comfortable. You will be instructed in the method to be used for keeping the abutments clean (see pages 59–65 of this booklet).

As with the stitches placed in your first surgery, those used to close the soft tissues during abutment connection will usually come out by themselves within 10 to 14 days. If not, or if a non-dissolving type of material is used, your dentist or surgeon will remove them.

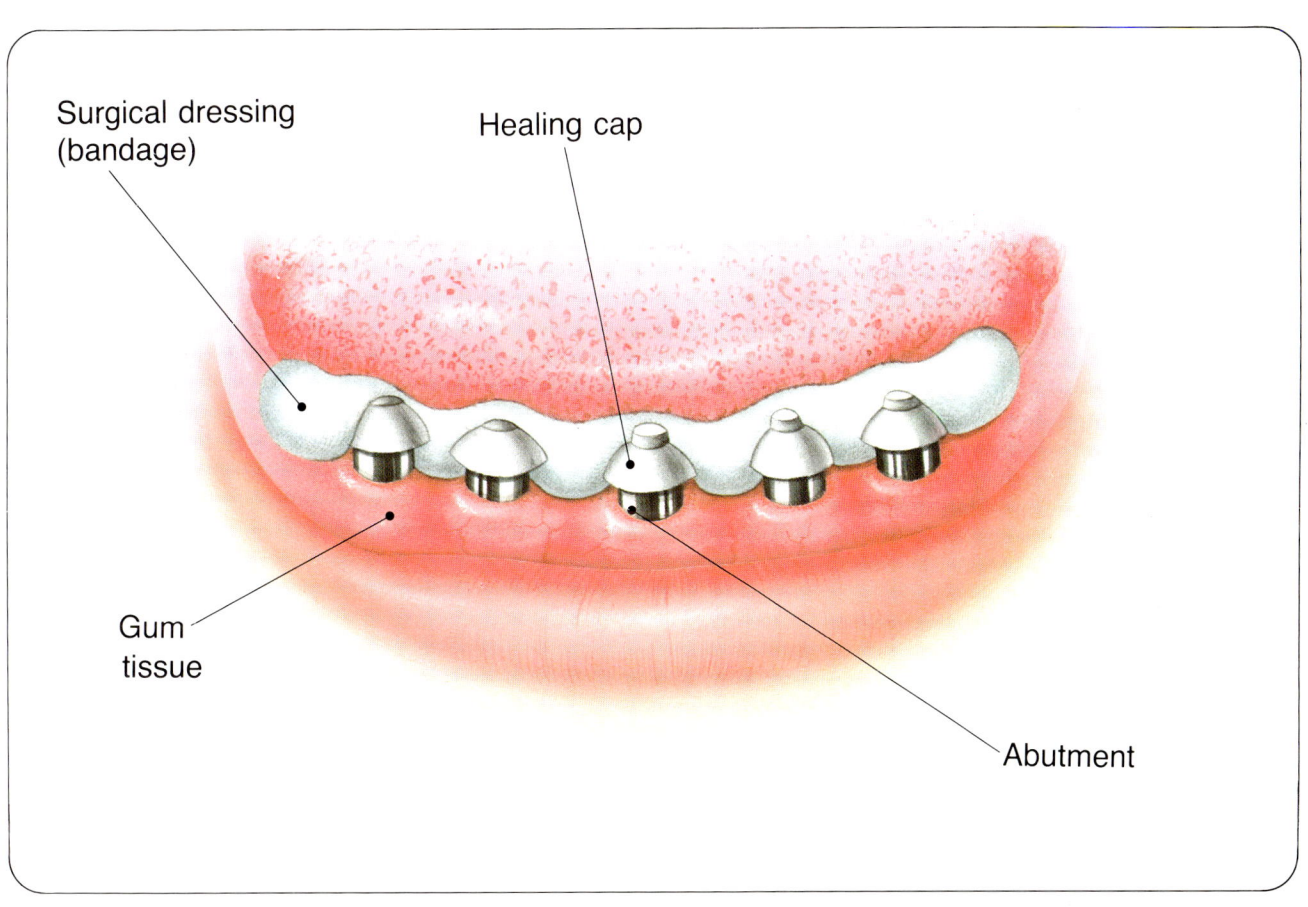

Restorative treatment

At least several days after the abutments have been attached to the integrated implants, impressions are again made of your mouth. Plaster-like models of the jaws and any teeth that you may still have can then be made from the impressions. The new replacement teeth (bridge or denture, also called a *prosthesis*) will eventually be made on these models.

If no natural teeth are present, bite records are made on temporary denture bases with wax rims. Artificial teeth are arranged on the bases so that the correct position of the teeth can be determined in your mouth.

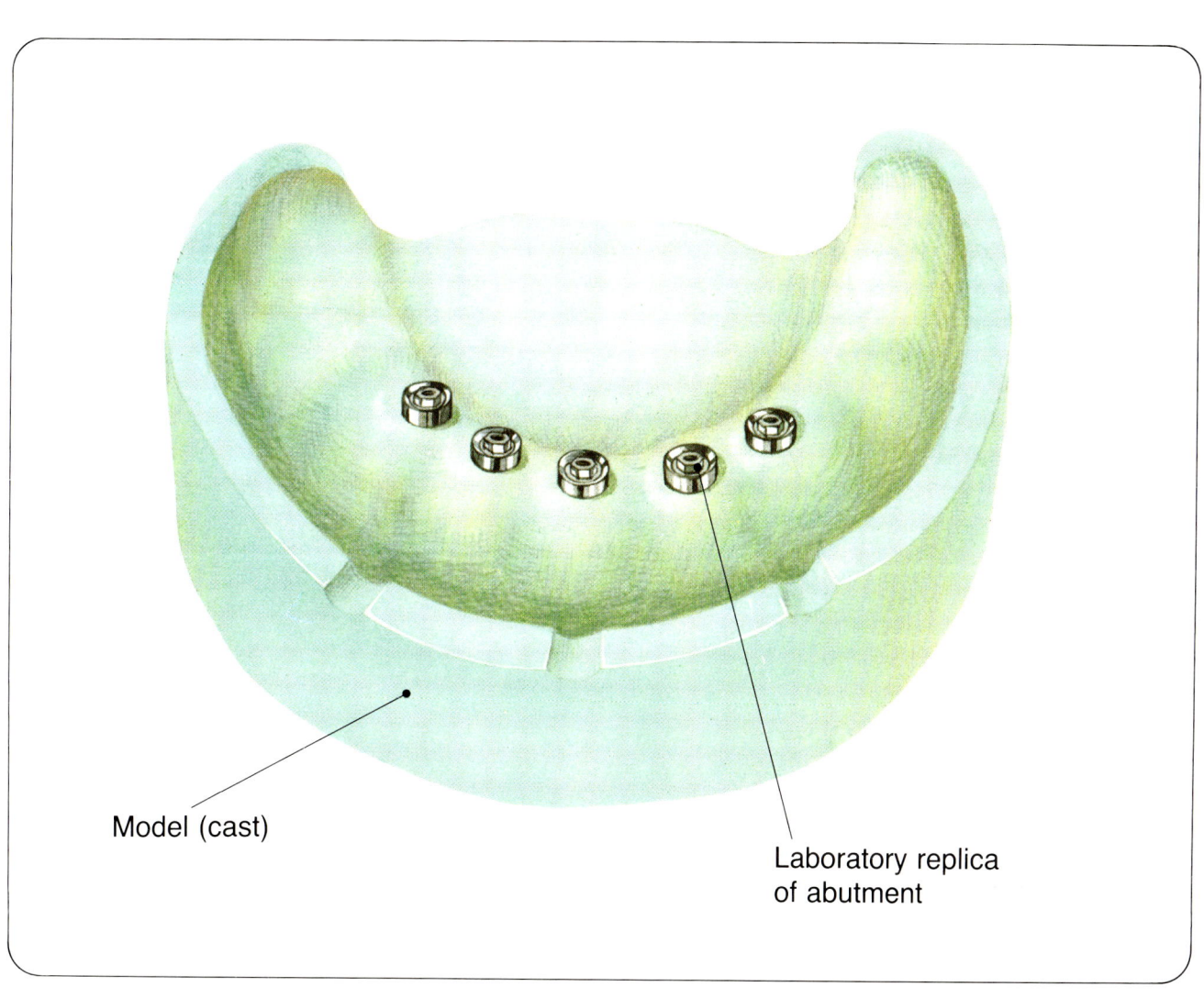

A metal framework is then made, and the artificial teeth are attached to this framework in the previously determined positions.

This whole assembly of framework and teeth will be tried in your mouth to see how it fits and looks. When the teeth look satisfactory and function properly, the prosthesis is completed.

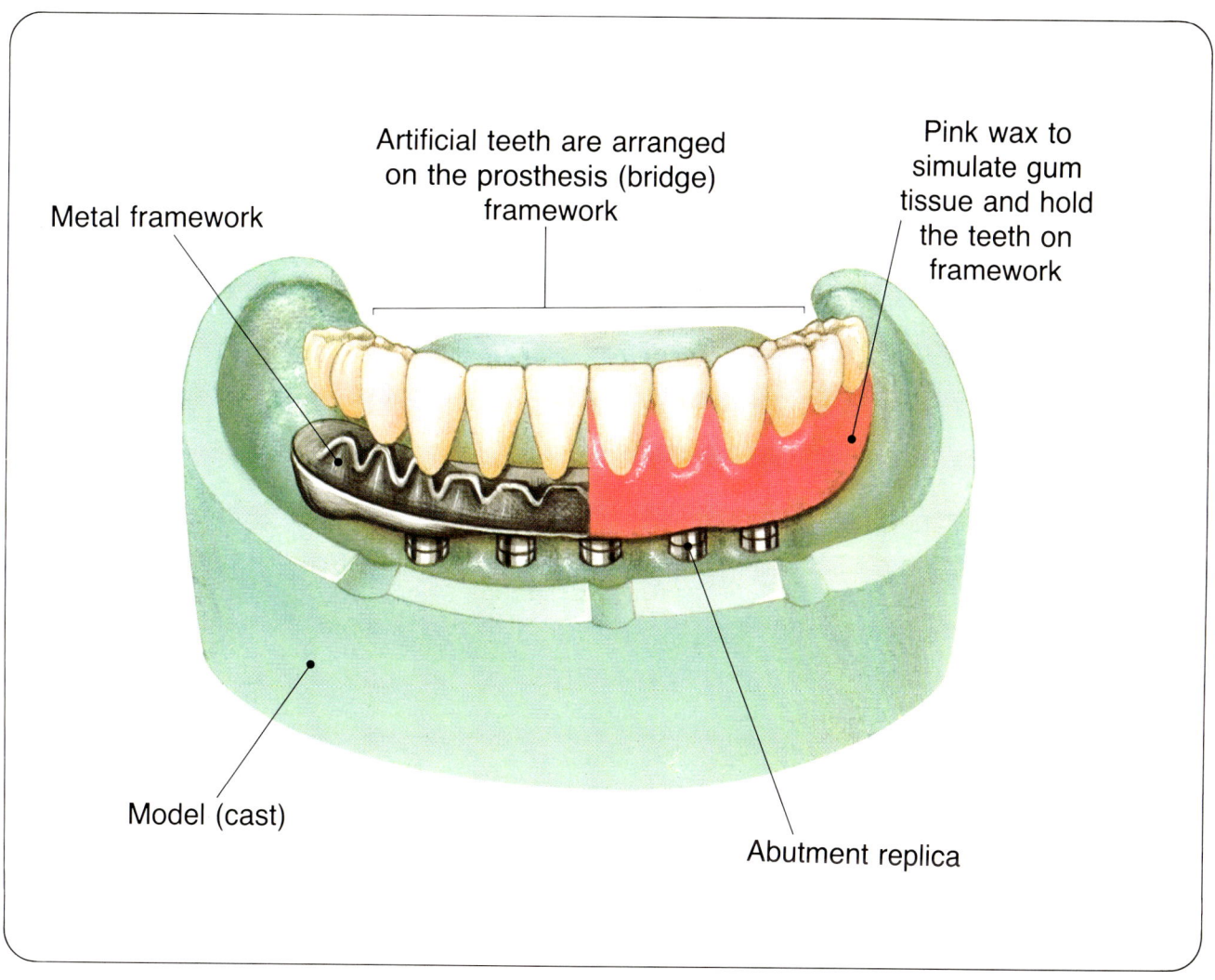

At last, the final prosthesis is secured on the abutments with small screws (or in situations where natural teeth also remain, with dental cement). This is called a **fixed prosthesis.**

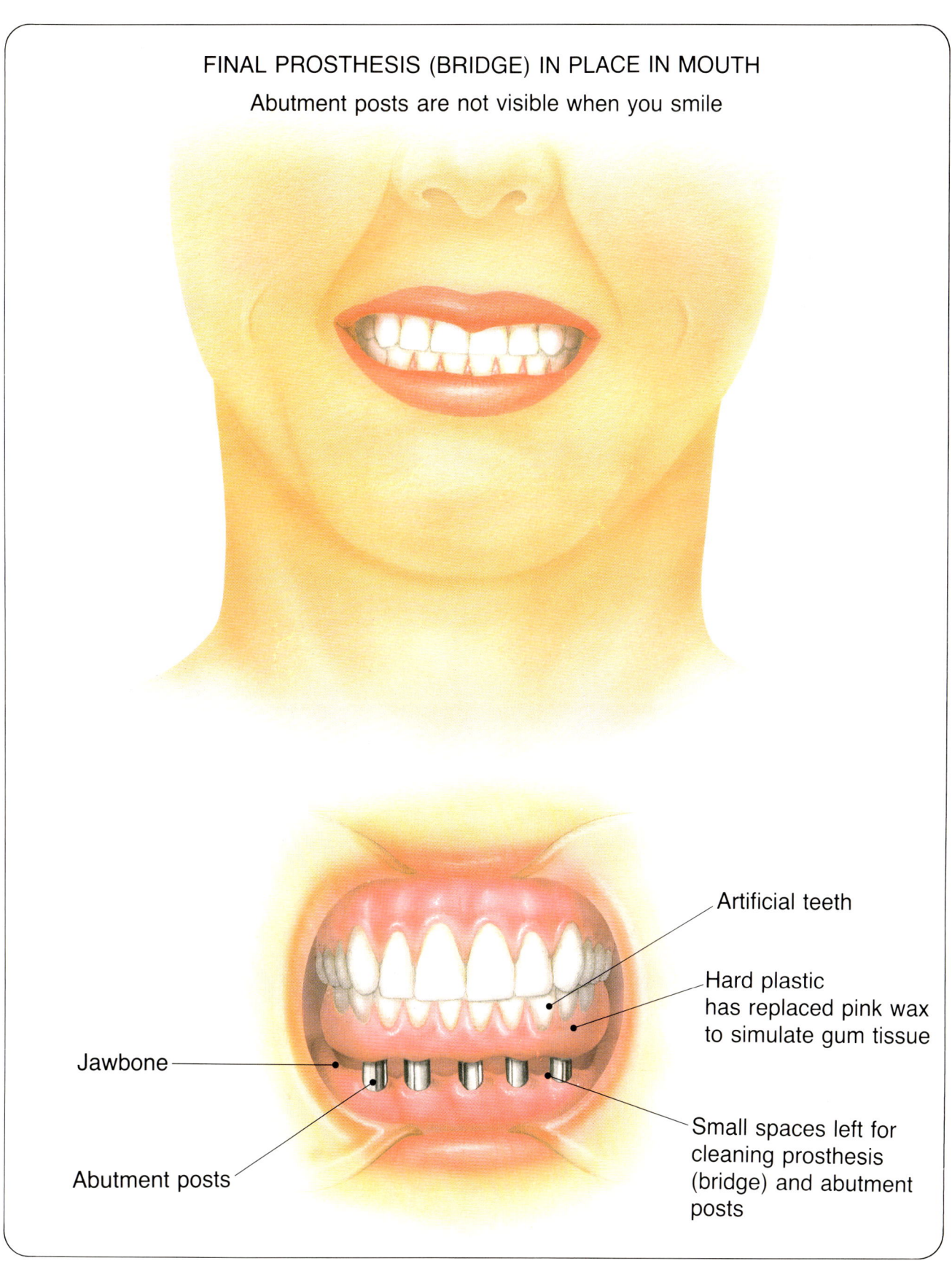

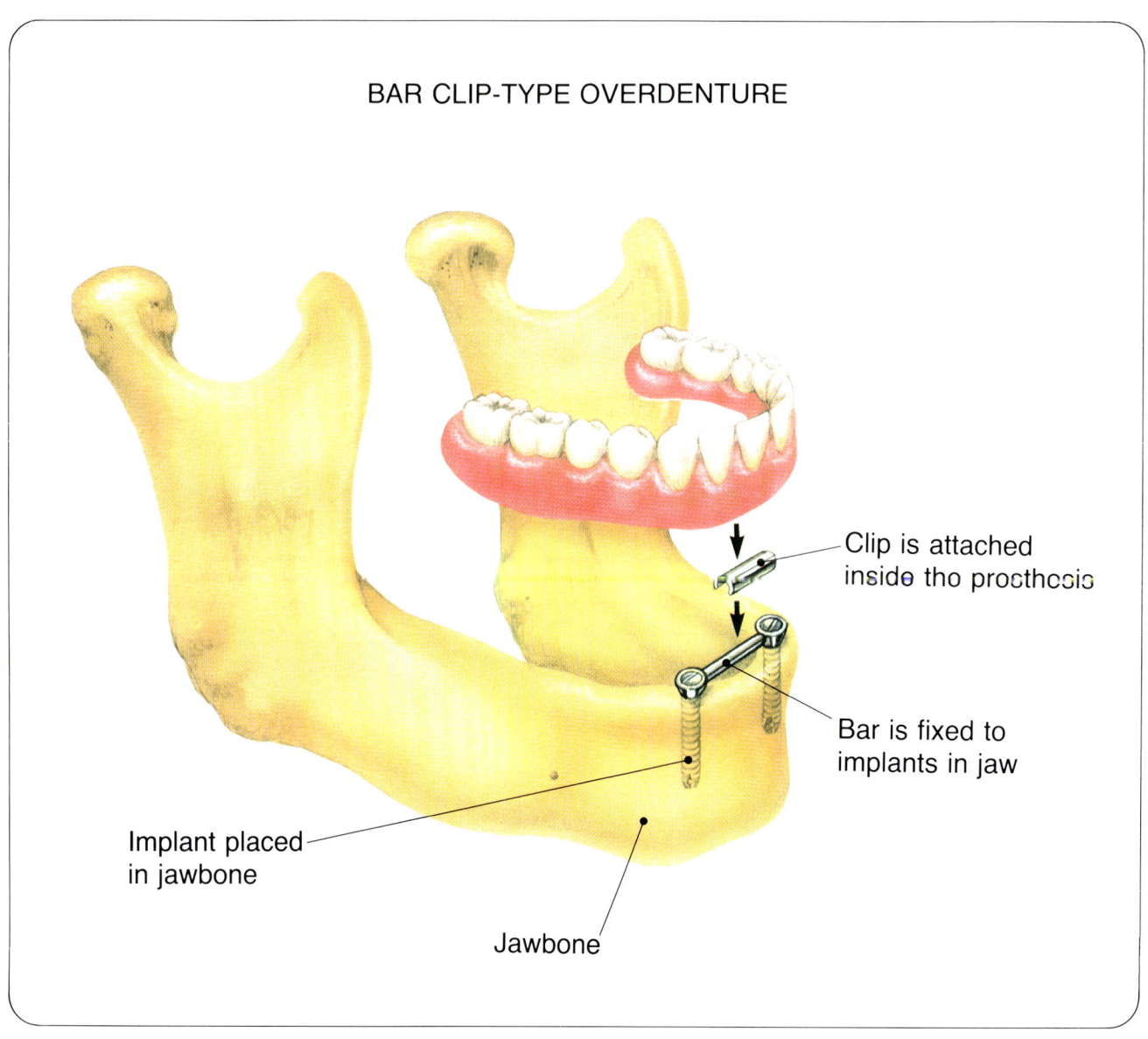

BAR CLIP-TYPE OVERDENTURE

- Clip is attached inside the prosthesis
- Bar is fixed to implants in jaw
- Implant placed in jawbone
- Jawbone

If it is not possible to construct a fixed prosthesis for your jaw, a removable overdenture may be designed to fit over the implants. While it is removable by you, it can be secured to the abutments by various types of attachments or magnets.

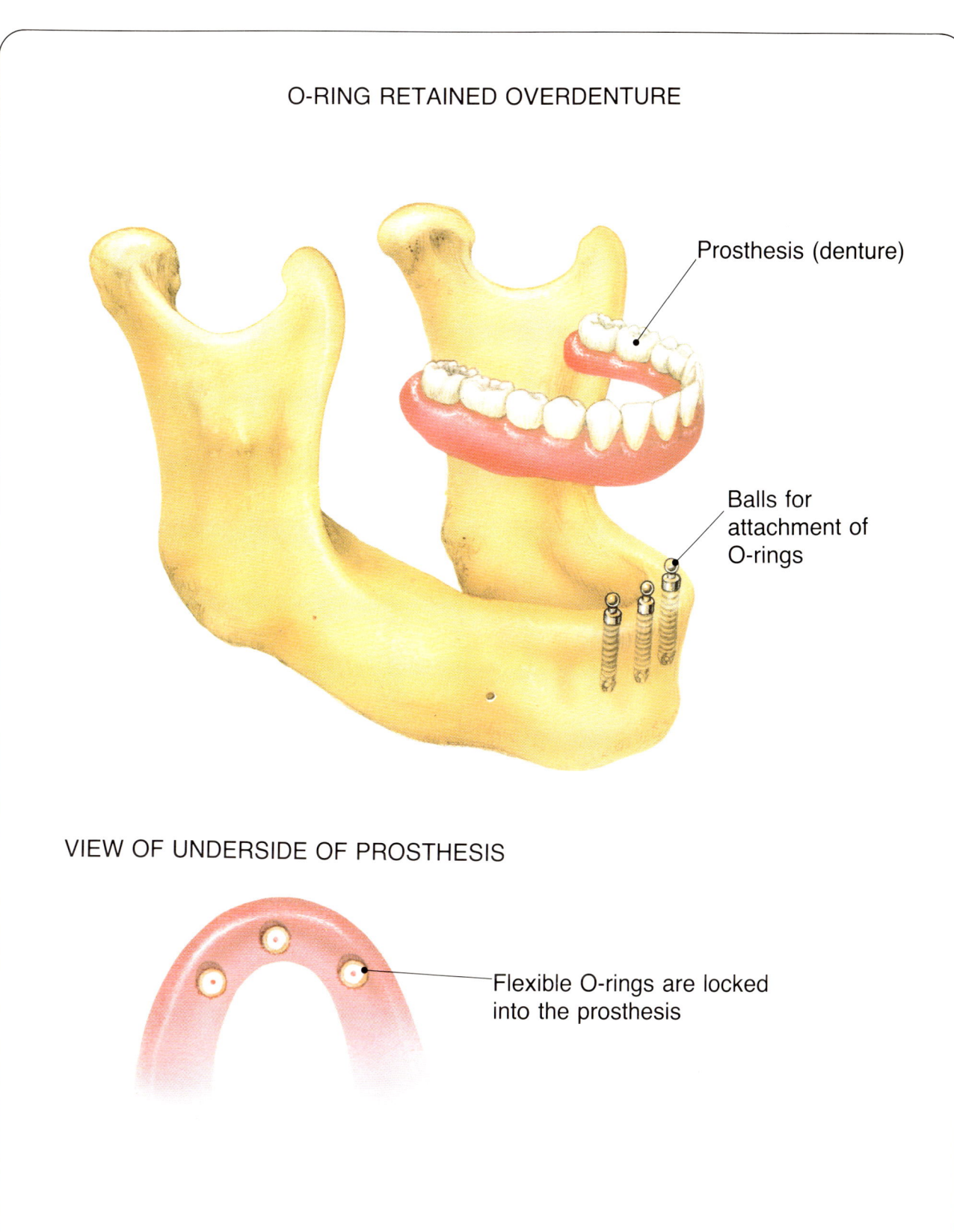

If you do have some remaining natural teeth, a prosthesis fixed to two or more implants may also be made to replace the missing teeth. They may be attached to natural teeth or may stand alone in the areas where teeth have been lost. Single missing teeth can be replaced by an implant-supported replacement tooth.

SINGLE-TOOTH REPLACEMENT

THREE-TOOTH PROSTHESIS

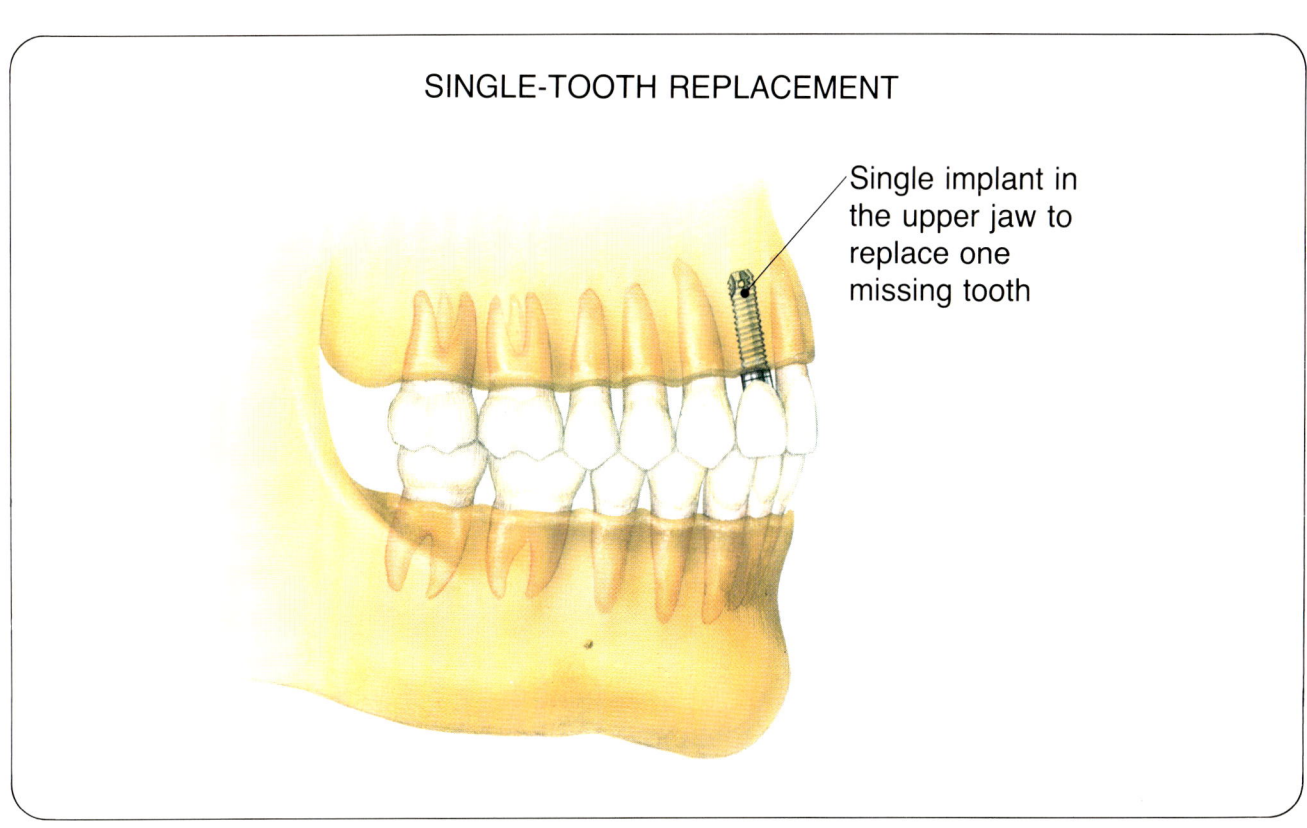

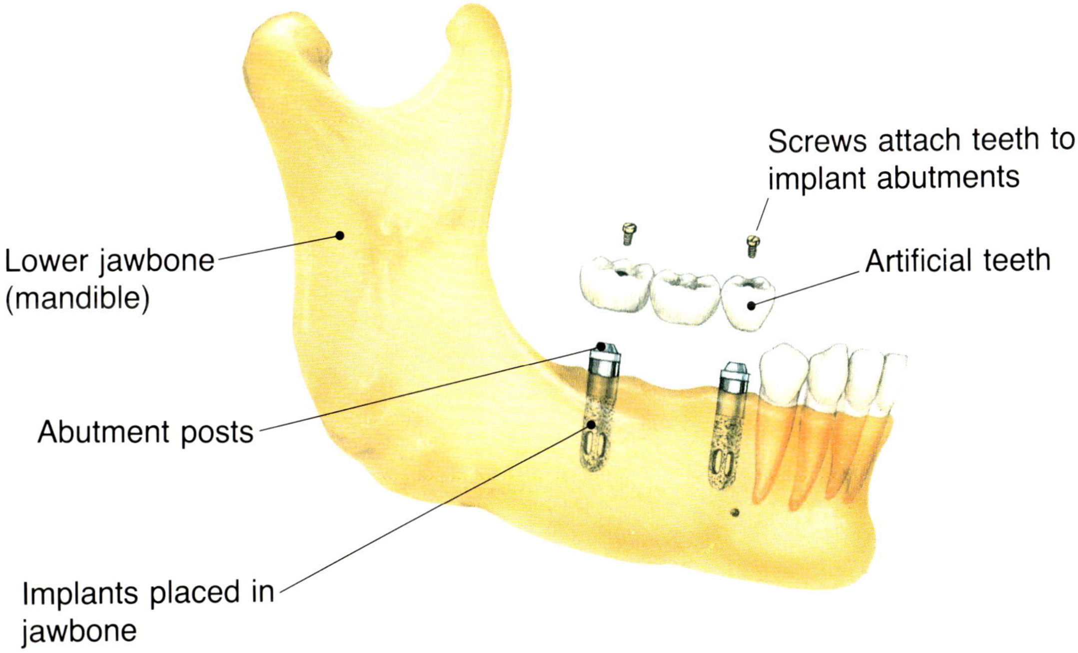

AFTERCARE

During the first year after your new prosthesis has been placed on the implants, it is necessary for the dentist to confirm that it fits well and works satisfactorily. Regular checkup appointments will usually be scheduled at 1-, 3-, and 6-month intervals in the first year. At these checkups, x-rays may be taken to examine the implant-bone relationship and rule out any disease. After the first year, follow-up examinations are usually necessary only once a year.

HOW TO CLEAN YOUR NEW TEETH AFTER IMPLANT THERAPY

Good oral hygiene is just as important to patients with an implant prosthesis as to those people who have their natural teeth. It cannot be said enough that you must thoroughly clean the abutments and prosthesis *daily* if your implants are to give you long-time service.

Because the flow of saliva slows down while you are asleep, the natural cleaning action of saliva decreases. This means that bacterial plaque builds up while you are asleep. Therefore, the most important times for cleaning the abutments and teeth are in the evening and in the morning.

The most important areas to be cleaned are the abutment posts, underneath the prosthesis, and the area around the gums. (The abutment posts, remember, are the shiny metal posts that stick up from the gums and attach the prosthesis to your jaw.)

Cleaning should be done in front of a large mirror with good lighting. A dental mirror (small round mirror on a handle) is helpful in seeing how well you have done the job. ▶

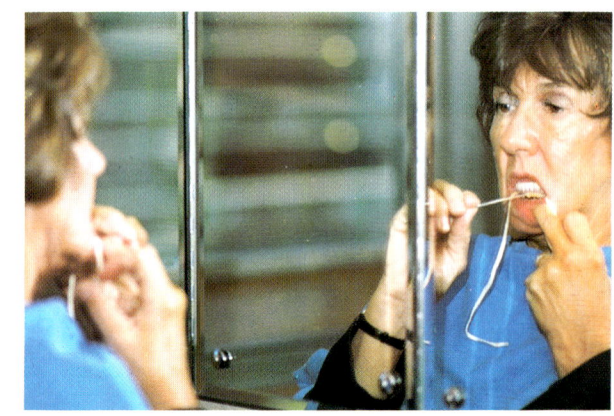

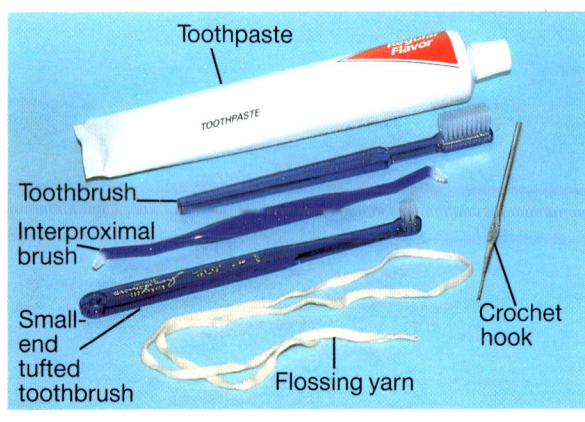

◀ Your dentist or dental assistant will show you how to find the right combination of cleaning techniques and instruments for your mouth.

FOLLOW THESE STEPS IN CLEANING YOUR
ABUTMENTS AND PROSTHESIS

1. Clean the abutment posts.

Clean the sides of the abutment posts and the undersurface of the prosthesis by passing cotton ribbon or thick floss through the space next to the abutment post, around the post, and then back out the front. ▶

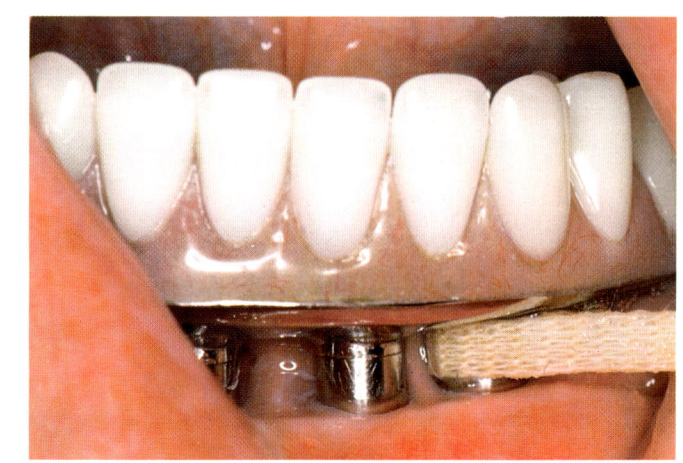

A crochet hook is very helpful in passing the ribbon through the space and then grasping it on the other side of the post to bring it forward.

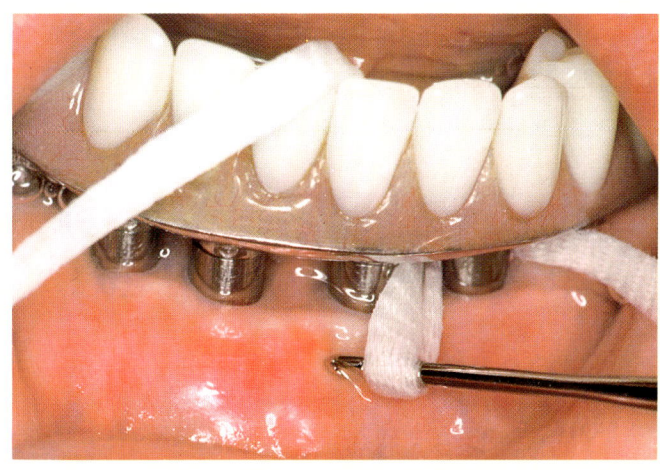

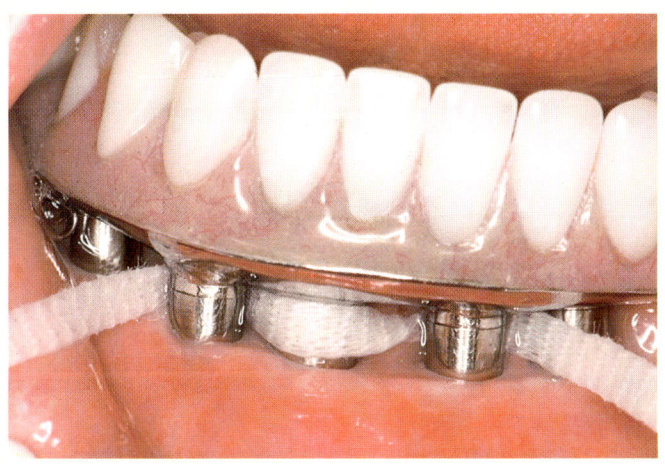

Or, you can wrap the ribbon around the posts in a figure eight (behind one post and in front of another post).

Then use the ribbon in the manner of a "shoe-shine rag" (a side-to-side motion) to polish the back and sides of the post from top to bottom. Many patients prefer to place toothpaste on the ribbon. It also provides a very mild abrasive that will help to polish the posts.

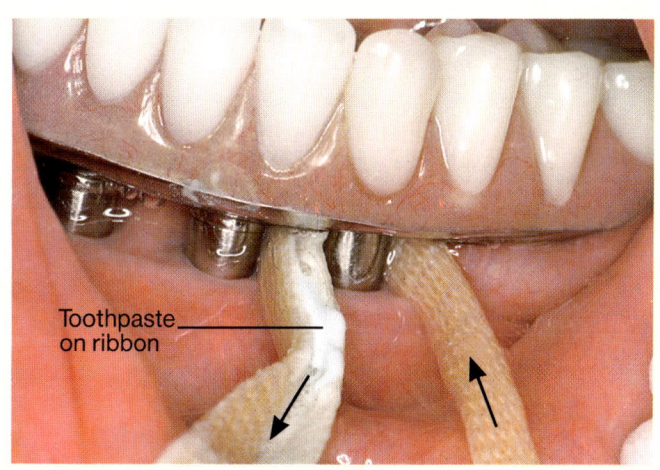

Toothpaste on ribbon

Follow these procedures for each post.

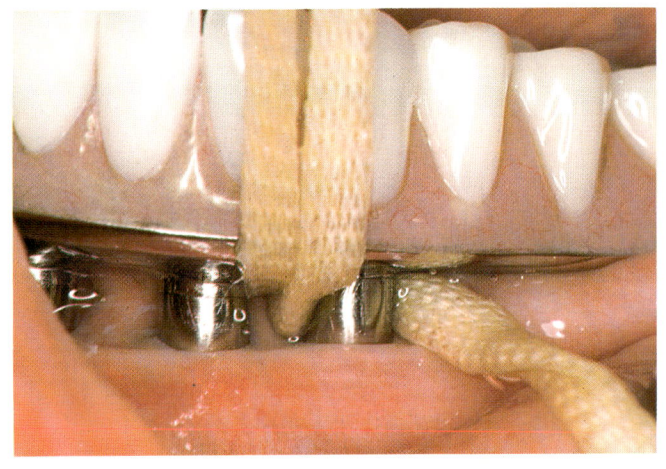

2. Clean the underside of the prosthesis.

◀ Use ribbon that has toothpaste on it to clean the *underside* of the prosthesis in each space. Use the ribbon again in the manner of a shoe-shine rag, but this time use a front to back stroke. Extra-thick floss is available at the drugstore and may also be used for this phase of cleaning.

Some patients find that an **interproximal** *("between surfaces")* **brush** helps in cleaning the sides of the abutment posts and the undersurface of the prosthesis. Use the brush with a back and forth stroke. ▶

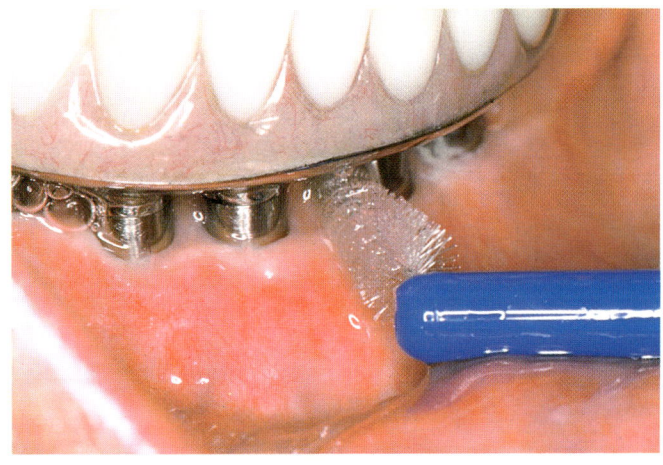

A small amount of toothpaste used with the brush may increase its ability to clean well.

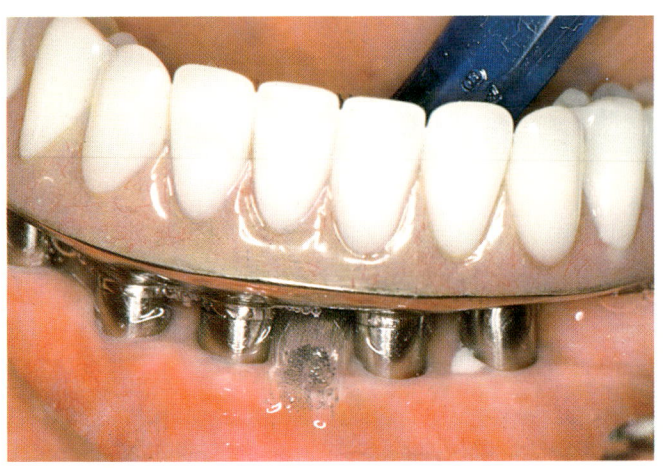

3. Brush the posts and prosthesis.

If you follow a set order each time you clean your prosthesis, as shown and described in the illustration, you will be sure that *all* surfaces will be clean.

Brush the upper and outer surfaces of the prosthesis as you would natural teeth, using a regular soft toothbrush.

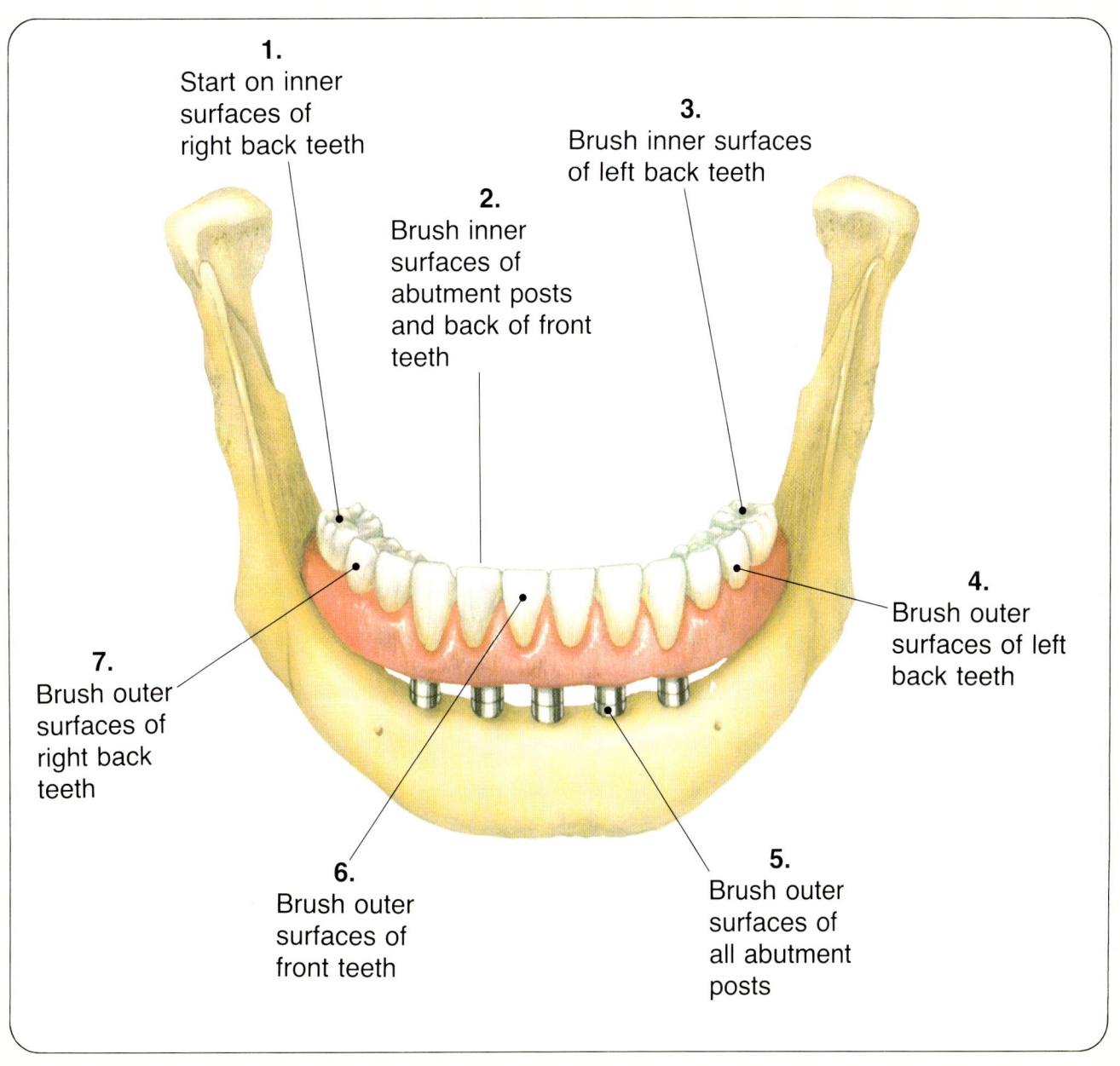

1. Start on inner surfaces of right back teeth
2. Brush inner surfaces of abutment posts and back of front teeth
3. Brush inner surfaces of left back teeth
4. Brush outer surfaces of left back teeth
5. Brush outer surfaces of all abutment posts
6. Brush outer surfaces of front teeth
7. Brush outer surfaces of right back teeth

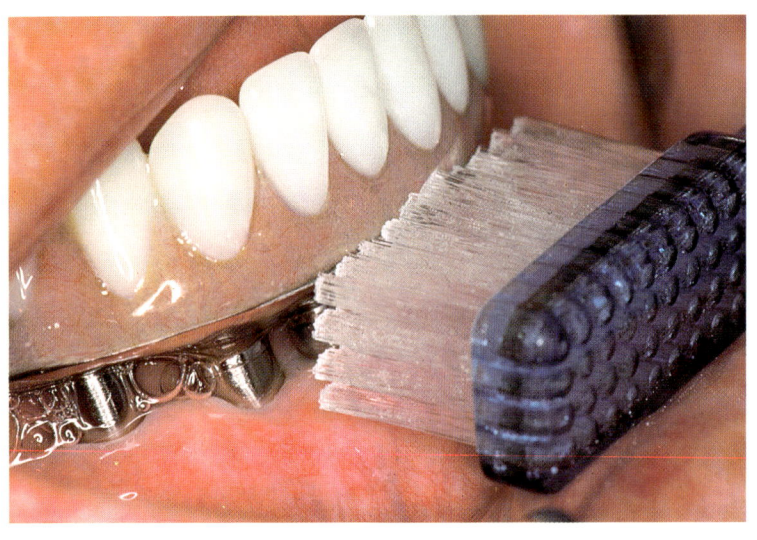

Clean the inner and outer sides of all abutment posts and surrounding gum tissues with a soft multi-tufted nylon toothbrush and toothpaste. Use a short, horizontal, back and forth movement. The brush is held at a 45 degree angle where the abutment post meets the gum tissue, as though you are intending to brush into a space between the gum tissues and the abutment post.

4. Rinse.

Finally, rinse your mouth thoroughly with water. Rinsing will remove the bacteria and food products that have been dislodged by your flossing and brushing. Some people prefer to rinse with a Water-Pik®; this is optional. It is important to remember that this device will not remove all plaque from the abutments or the prosthesis.

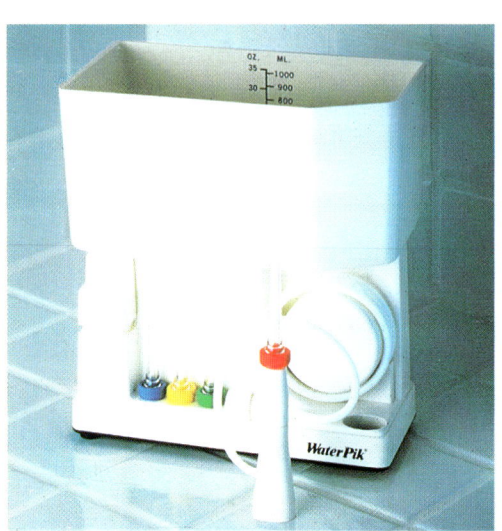

The Water-Pik® can be used to *supplement* the brushing and flossing but it is not a substitute for them. ▶

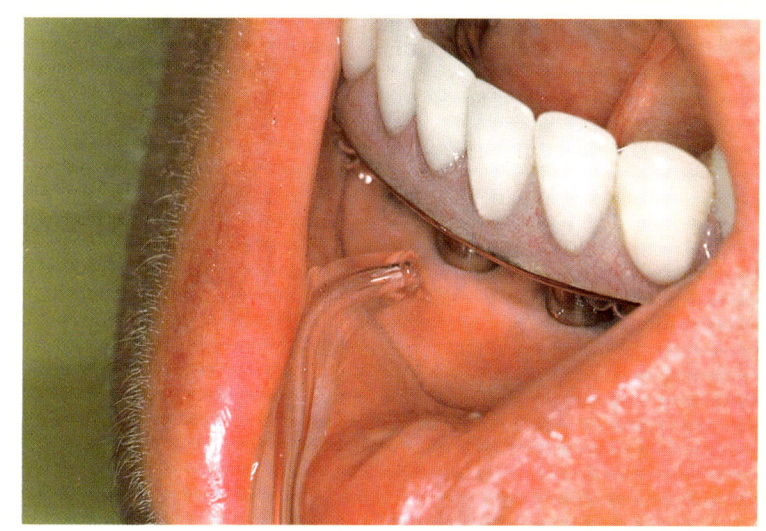

If you have a removable prosthesis:

A removable overdenture is usually cleaned in the same manner as above. However, because the materials in an overdenture vary, your dentist will instruct you on how to care for it.

Don't get frustrated—With practice you will improve your cleaning technique!

And remember: when you clean your abutments, prosthesis, and gums every day, you can prevent inflammation of the gums. This means:

- You can prevent loss of bone around the implants
- Your prosthesis will remain secured
- You will be able to chew well and comfortably and smile with confidence!

THINGS TO REMEMBER

Implants are a relatively new type of dental treatment. Today they appear to be a very successful answer to the problem of missing teeth. As with any type of medical care, there is no guarantee for 100% success for all patients. Your dentist will be able to give you an idea about how successful the implant system selected for you has been. It is important for you to realize that some implants fail and have to be removed. The rate of failure for different implant systems varies from less than 1% to 40%–50%. Your individual chances for successful implant treatment should be carefully explained by your dentist before you begin treatment.

Successful implant treatment has dramatically improved the quality of life for many people. With proper planning and care, implants can be an excellent answer to the problems associated with missing natural teeth.

HOW TO CLEAN YOUR NEW TEETH AFTER IMPLANT THERAPY

Good oral hygiene is just as important to patients with an implant prosthesis as to those people who have their natural teeth. It cannot be said enough that you must thoroughly clean the abutments and prosthesis *daily* if your implants are to give you long-time service.

Because the flow of saliva slows down while you are asleep, the natural cleaning action of saliva decreases. This means that bacterial plaque builds up while you are asleep. Therefore, the most important times for cleaning the abutments and teeth are in the evening and in the morning.

The most important areas to be cleaned are the abutment posts, underneath the prosthesis, and the area around the gums. (The abutment posts, remember, are the shiny metal posts that stick up from the gums and attach the prosthesis to your jaw.)

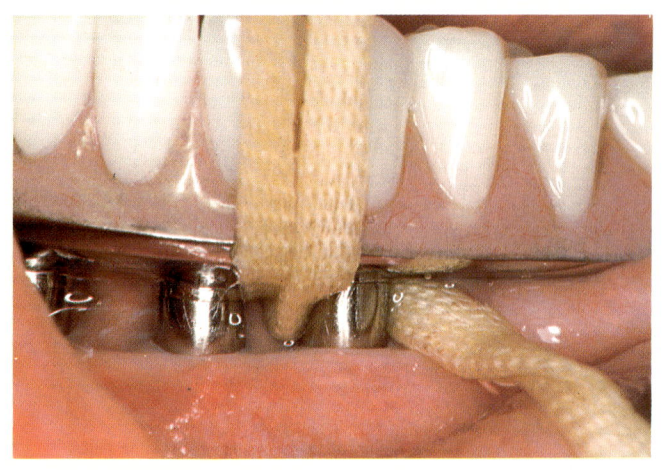

2. Clean the underside of the prosthesis.

◀ Use ribbon that has toothpaste on it to clean the *underside* of the prosthesis in each space. Use the ribbon again in the manner of a shoe-shine rag, but this time use a front to back stroke. Extra-thick floss is available at the drugstore and may also be used for this phase of cleaning.

Some patients find that an **interproximal** *("between surfaces")* **brush** helps in cleaning the sides of the abutment posts and the undersurface of the prosthesis. Use the brush with a back and forth stroke. ▶

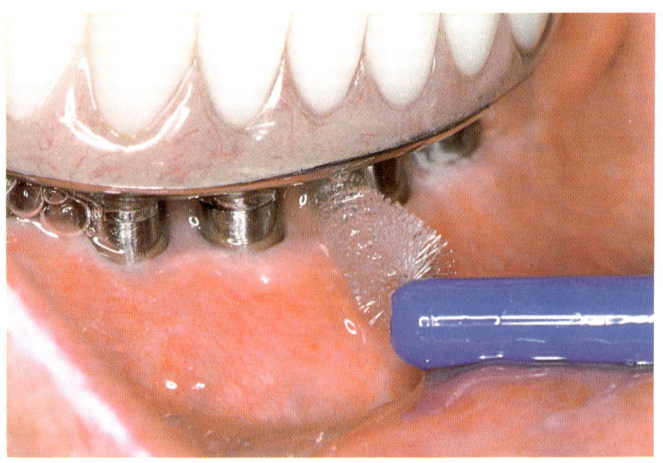

A small amount of toothpaste used with the brush may increase its ability to clean well.

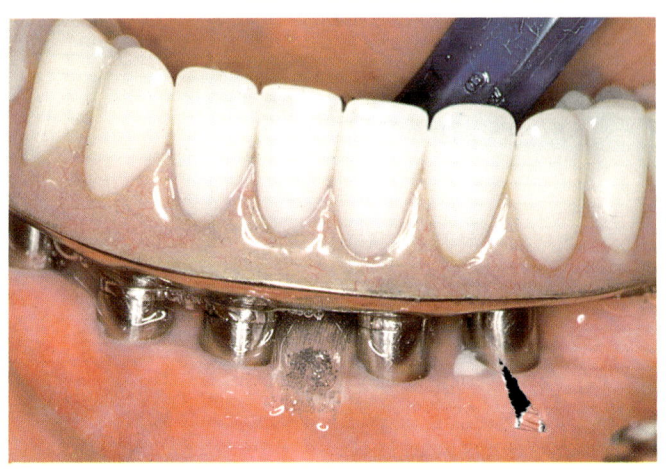

A crochet hook is very helpful in passing the ribbon through the space and then grasping it on the other side of the post to bring it forward.

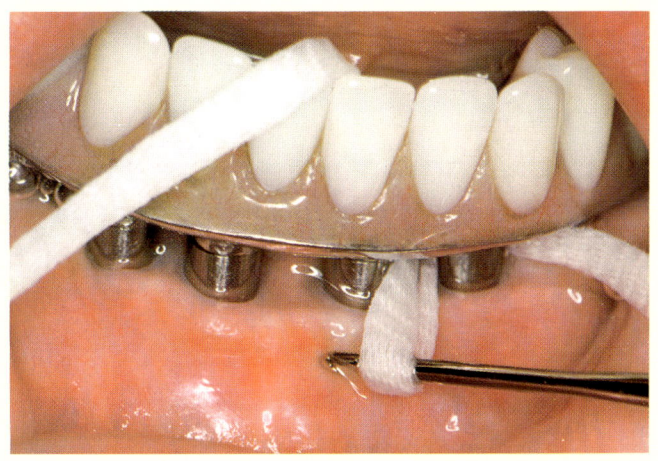

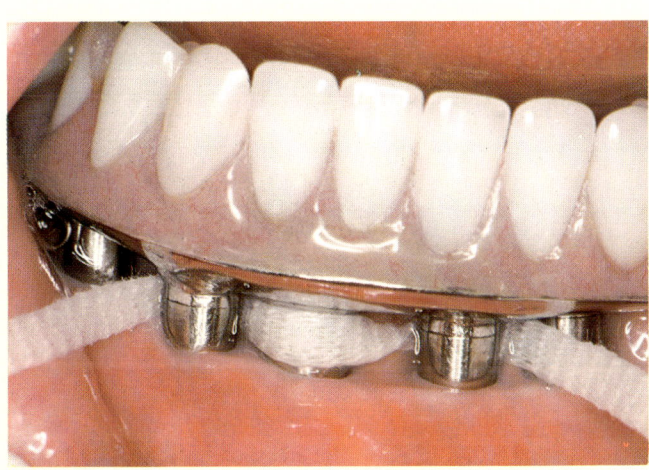

Or, you can wrap the ribbon around the posts in a figure eight (behind one post and in front of another post).

Then use the ribbon in the manner of a "shoe-shine rag" (a side-to-side motion) to polish the back and sides of the post from top to bottom. Many patients prefer to place toothpaste on the ribbon. It also provides a very mild abrasive that will help to polish the posts.

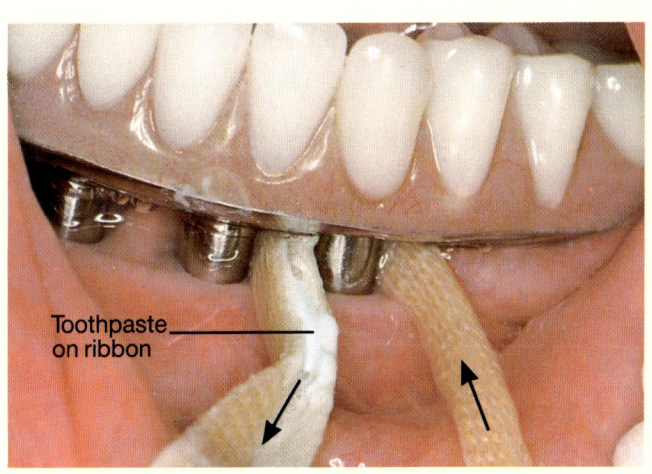

Toothpaste on ribbon

Follow these procedures for each post.

3

Cleaning should be done in front of a large mirror with good lighting. A dental mirror (small round mirror on a handle) is helpful in seeing how well you have done the job.

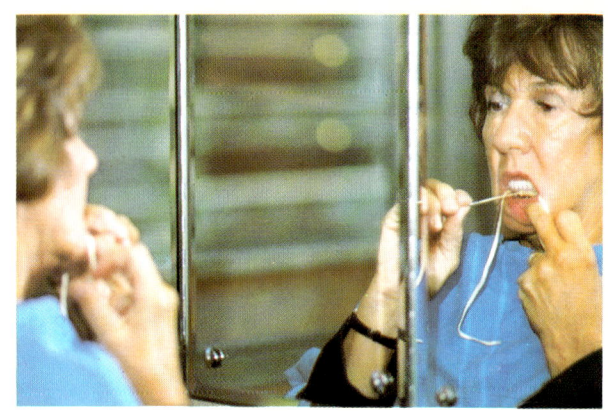

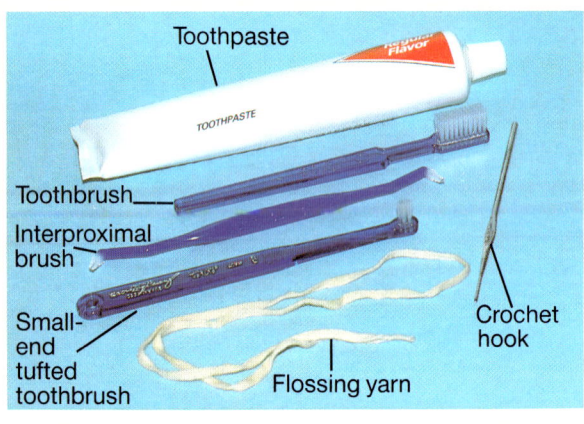

Your dentist or dental assistant will show you how to find the right combination of cleaning techniques and instruments for your mouth.

FOLLOW THESE STEPS IN CLEANING YOUR ABUTMENTS AND PROSTHESIS

1. Clean the abutment posts.

Clean the sides of the abutment posts and the undersurface of the prosthesis by passing cotton ribbon or thick floss through the space next to the abutment post, around the post, and then back out the front.

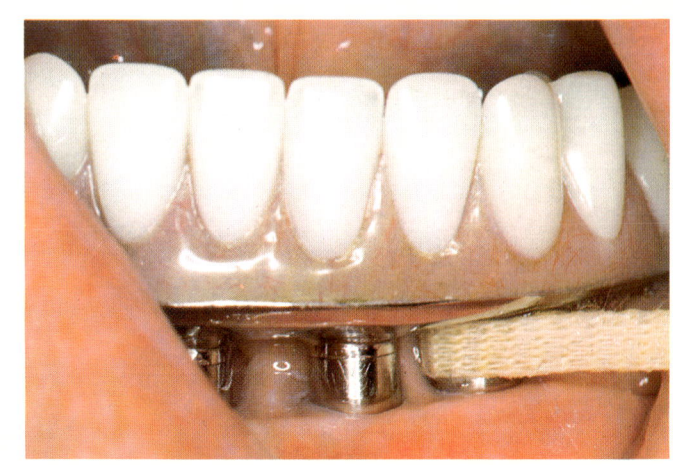

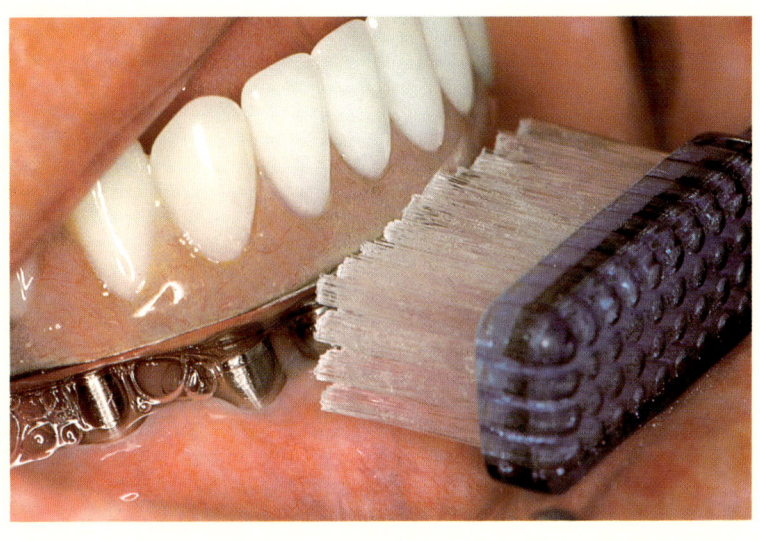

Clean the inner and outer sides of all abutment posts and surrounding gum tissues with a soft multi-tufted nylon toothbrush and toothpaste. Use a short, horizontal, back and forth movement. The brush is held at a 45 degree angle where the abutment post meets the gum tissue, as though you are intending to brush into a space between the gum tissues and the abutment post.

4. Rinse.

Finally, rinse your mouth thoroughly with water. Rinsing will remove the bacteria and food products that have been dislodged by your flossing and brushing. Some people prefer to rinse with a Water-Pik®; this is optional. It is important to remember that this device will not remove all plaque from the abutments or the prosthesis.

▼

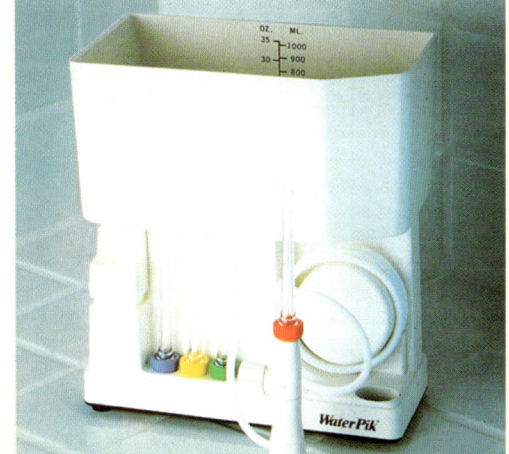

6

The Water-Pik® can be used to *supplement* the brushing and flossing but it is not a substitute for them. ▶

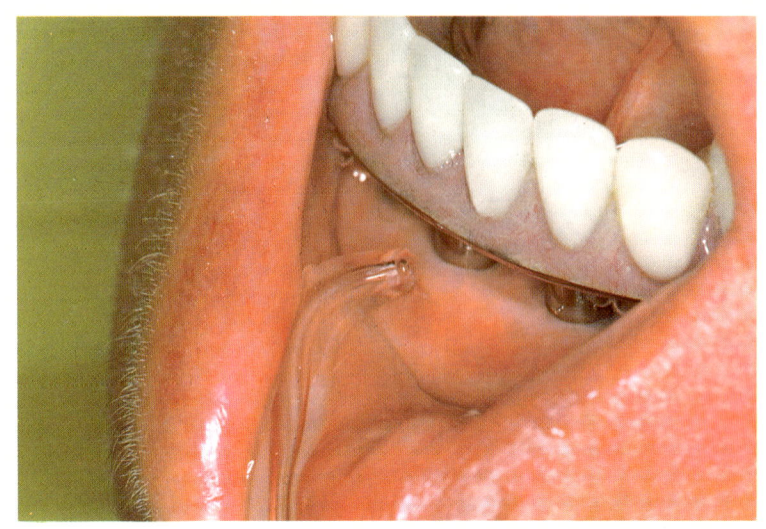

If you have a removable prosthesis:

A removable overdenture is usually cleaned in the same manner as above. However, because the materials in an overdenture vary, your dentist will instruct you on how to care for it.

Don't get frustrated—With practice you will improve your cleaning technique!

And remember: when you clean your abutments, prosthesis, and gums every day, you can prevent inflammation of the gums. This means:

- You can prevent loss of bone around the implants
- Your prosthesis will remain secured
- You will be able to chew well and comfortably and smile with confidence!

Special instructions:

```
┌─────────────────────────────────────────────┐
│                                             │
│         FUTURE APPOINTMENT SCHEDULE         │
│                                             │
│    Date                              Time   │
│    _____      │
│                                             │
│    _____      │
│                                             │
│    _____      │
│                                             │
│    _____      │
│                                             │
│    _____      │
│                                             │
└─────────────────────────────────────────────┘
```

Your dentist is:

3. Brush the posts and prosthesis.

If you follow a set order each time you clean your prosthesis, as shown and described in the illustration, you will be sure that *all* surfaces will be clean.

Brush the upper and outer surfaces of the prosthesis as you would natural teeth, using a regular soft toothbrush.

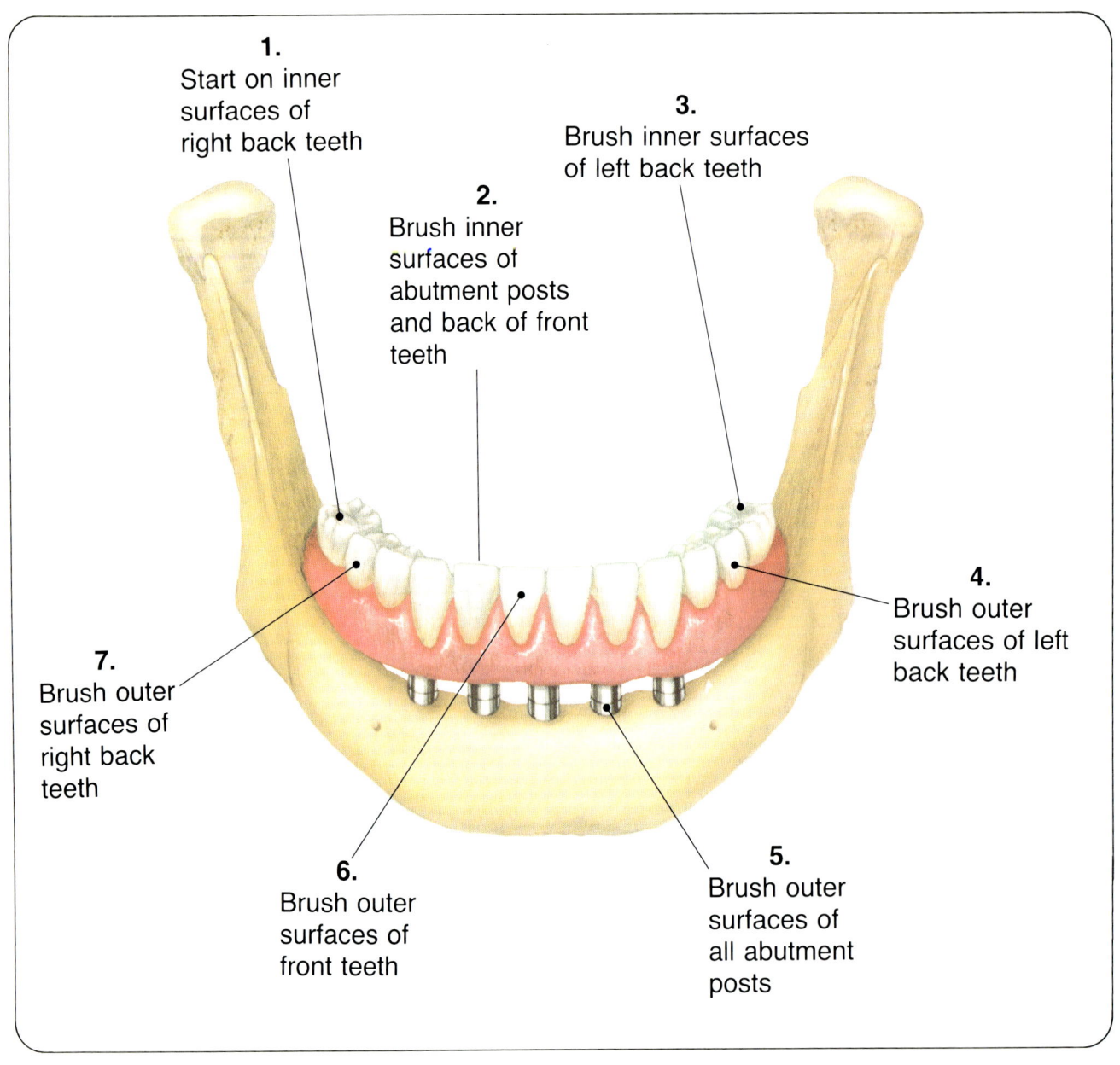

1. Start on inner surfaces of right back teeth

2. Brush inner surfaces of abutment posts and back of front teeth

3. Brush inner surfaces of left back teeth

4. Brush outer surfaces of left back teeth

5. Brush outer surfaces of all abutment posts

6. Brush outer surfaces of front teeth

7. Brush outer surfaces of right back teeth